Manual of Veterinary Entomology & Acarology

S.K. Gupta
Rajinder Kumar
Department of Veterinary Parasitology
College of Veterinary Sciences
CCS Haryana Agricultural Univesity
Hisar - 125 004, Haryana, INDIA

IBDC
International Book Distributing Co.
(Publishing Division)

Published by

INTERNATIONAL BOOK DISTRIBUTING CO.
(Publishing Division)
Chaman Studio Building, 2nd Floor,
Charbagh, Lucknow 226 004 U.P. (INDIA)
Tel. : Off. : 2450004, 2450007, 2459058 Fax : 0522-2458629
E-Mail : ibdco@sancharnet.in

First Edition. 2003

Price: Rs. 140/-

ISBN 81-85860-85-8

Composed & Designed at :

Panacea Computers
33, Nehru Road,
Sadar Cantt. Lucknow-226 002
Phone : 2481164, 2480546
E-mail : prasgupt@rediffmail.com

Printed at:

Army Printing Press
33, Nehru Road,
Sadar Cantt. Lucknow-226 002
Phone : 2481164, 2480546, Fax : 0522-2480543
E-mail : armypress@indiatimes.com

Preface

Veterinary Entomology and Acarology deal with the arthropods affecting livestock and poultry. Arthropods are included in the largest phylum, Arthropoda of the animal kingdom. They show a great diversity in their morphology, habitat, habits, development etc. and constitute about more than 80 percent of total animal population in the world. They produce harmful effects through their direct pestilence (blood sucking, painful bites, irritation, annoyance, gadding, maggot wound etc.) as well as being vector of disease pathogens (helminths, protozoa, rickettsia, bacteria and viruses). For their effective control a definitive diagnosis is required for which their identification is essential.

The intent of this manual is to provide an aid in the diagnosis of important arthropods of veterinary and medical importance to the students, teachers and field veterinarians. This manual contains not only the arthropod parasites included in the course contents devised by Veterinary Council of India but also others, which have their importance in Veterinary Medicine.

In this manual, we have given the detailed morphological description of adult arthropods as well as their developing stages along with the illustrations for better understanding the diagnostic features. Additionally, the commonly used techniques in Entomology have also been incorporated. The economic importance of each arthropod has also been described to make the readers understand their role as direct pestilence or vectors of various diseases of domestic animals, birds and human-beings.

We hope that this manual will be of considerable help to the students and teachers of Veterinary Colleges, all over India as well as to the field veterinarians.

Last but not the least, the constant encouragement given by our present Dean, Dr. A.P. Singh for preparing practical manuals for all the courses is highly appreciable.

Authors

CONTENTS

Topic	Page No.

Topic	Page No.

1. GENERAL CHARACTERS OF ARTHROPODS

The word arthropod is of Greek origin and consists of two parts i.e. arthro : joint + podus : foot or appendage. Phylum Arthropoda represents invertebrates having jointed appendages, bilateral symmetry, an exoskeleton; triploblastic body with metameric segmentation (18-22 segments); striated muscles; open circulatory system; chewing, sucking or non-functional mouth parts with lateral jaws; respiration by gills, tracheae, lung books or body surface; excretion by coxal gland or Malpighian tubules; sexes separate (except in some of the crustaceans); nervous system with paired ganglia; sensory organs like antennae, brain, eyes, bristles etc. In-spite of these similarities, it comprises the most diverse and the largest group of animals having more than 80% species of all the known animals.

Body : Basically, the insect body is divisible into head, which has about 6 fused segments; thorax, which has 3 segments viz., prothorax, mesothorax and metathorax from front to posterior region; and abdomen, which has 11 segments. Head carries the antennae, eyes, mouthparts and brain; thorax carries legs corresponding to thoracic segments, and the wings; abdomen carries reproductive organs, and major part of gut enclosed in the body cavity (haemocoel). The place where various parts joint, is termed suture, which is clearer in embryological state than afterwards.

Cuticle : Morphologically, the cuticle is laminated and consists of epicuticle, procuticle (exocuticle + endocuticle) and hypodermis (also referred as epidermis). The cuticle may be smooth, notched, pitted, ridged or spinose in its character.

Sclerite : The exoskeleton is usually present in the form of plates called sclerites. They are delimited by sutures or membranous areas.

Tagma : Fusion of segments to form definite regions like thorax, abdomen etc.

Tergum : Dorsal sclerite is called tergum (pl. tergite). The tergite are transversely elongated, overlapping plates. Each plate overlaps its successor.

Sternum : Ventral sclerite is called sternum (pl. sternite). The sternite are transversely elongated, overlapping plates. In the higher DIPTERA, the sternite are greatly reduced.

Pleuron : A lateral plate between tergum and sternum is called pleuron.

Antennae : They are sense organs and are tactile (feelers) or olfactory in function. They exist in the form of two or more mobile articulation appendages. The antennae may be : **Setiform :** Bristle shaped, tapering apically by reduction in the diameter of the segments e.g. Coleoptera, Diptera and Lepidoptera; **Filiform :** Threadlike, segments of nearly equal diameter e.g. Orthoptera, some of the Coleoptera and Lepidoptera; **Moniliform :** Necklace type, have series of globular beads e.g. Coleoptera : **Pectinate :** Comb like having fine feather like processes; **Clavate :** Club shaped, in which segments increase in diameter apically e.g. Hemiptera, Hymenoptera, etc.; **Aristate :** The large terminal portion ends in seta or bears an appendage which is hair like and is called arista. In some insects the antennae show sexual dimorphism i.e. plumose in males and pilose in females.

Arista : The third segment of antenna may be enlarged and possesses a bristly outgrowth at its base called arista.

Legs : They are hollow cylindrical outgrowths or continuations of body, which arise at the junctions of pleura and sterna. Various parts from proximal to distal end of the leg are : Coxa, trochanter, femur, tibia and tarsus. All the five parts are capable of independent movement and show slight modification from insect to insect. The number of legs and their parts are uniform in a particular taxonomic group.

Ecdysis : The casting off of the exoskeleton in the life phases of arthropods is called ecdysis (moulting/molting). Ecdysis helps to accommodate the growing tissues.

Tracheae : They constitute a ventilation system of air tubes ramifying all through the body.

Spiracles : The external openings of tracheae are called spiracles.

Haemocoel : The body cavity of arthropods is full of blood and is called haemocoel.

Circulatory system : It is poorly developed and consists of contractile pipe and an open portion, haemocoel.

Chaetotaxy : It is that branch of Entomology, which deals with the study of bristles. In a number of cases, chaetotaxy forms the basis of classification.

Metamorphosis : A change in the form of arthropods associated with ecdysis is called metamorphosis; each form thus produced is called instar. Following types of metamorphosis are recognized:

a) **Ametabola :** The arthropods of this group show no or negligible metamorphosis. It exists in the primitive type of insects e.g. silverfish.

b) **Hemimetabola :** This group of arthropods show slight

metamorphosis (incomplete metamorphosis) e.g. cockroaches, grasshoppers, lice, bed bugs etc. The young ones coming out of eggs are called nymphs, which resemble to a great extent with the adults.

c) **Holometabola :** This group of arthropods shows complete metamorphosis. The different stages encountered are egg – larva – pupa – adult e.g. *Musca, Stomoxys, Tabanus* etc.

Wings : Some insects have two pairs of wings, first pair being mesothoracic and second one metathoracic in origin. In Diptera, the second pair of wings is reduced to slender knob-like structures called halters. Grossly, the wing has 4 parts viz. squama, antisquama, alula, and wing proper. It varies in shape, size and is roughly triangular. Anterior margin is called costa, posterior one, anal and the outer one as apical (Plate:I).

Wing venation : The wing veins are actually tracheae through which the blood circulates in the nymphal or pupal stage which may continue for sometime even in the adult stage. There is a set pattern of wing venation in a species, which helps in classification and identification. Wing has longitudinal and cross veins. (Plate : I). The six longitudinal veins running one behind the other are as follows :

1. **Costa :** It runs along the anterior margin and is unbranched.
2. **Subcosta :** It is located behind the costa and may rarely be branched.
3. **Radius :** It runs behind the subcosta and has five branches named R_1, R_2, R_3, R_4 and R_5, respectively. A fusion in these branches may be there.
4. **Media :** It runs behind the radius and divides into two

branches, which further subdivide in M_1, M_2, M_3 and M_4.

5. **Cubitus :** It is located behind the media and divides into two branches namely Cu_1 and Cu_2.

6. **Anal veins :** They are usually two in number called A_1 and A_2.

Cross veins : The cross veins delineate areas of wings called cells. Various cross veins are :

1. **Humeral cross vein :** It extends from the costa to the subcosta near the humeral angle of the wing.

2. **Radio-medial cross vein :** It connects radius with the media near the middle of the wing.

3. **Medial cross vein :** It runs between the branches of M_2 and M_3 of the media.

4. **Medio-cubital cross vein :** It connects media with the cubitus.

The cells formed are named after the longitudinal veins that form the anterior margin of the cell. If a cell is completely closed by the veins, it is called closed cell. If it extends towards the outer margin, it is called open cell. A cell formed at the apex of the wing is called apical cell and a cell surrounded from all sides by veins is called discal cell.

Digestive system : Digestive tract is not uniform in all the classes of arthropods but mostly they possess a complete alimentary tract, which begins with the mouth at the anterior part and ends at the anus on the posterior part. Besides the alimentary canal, there are other associated organs like a pair of lobed salivary glands, gastric caeca and Malpighian tubules. The alimentary canal is an asymmetrical tube oriented lengthwise in the body cavity and consists of three parts :

1. Stomodaeum (Foregut)
2. Mesenteron (Midgut/ventriculus)
3. Proctodaeum (Hindgut)

The stomodaeum includes mouth, pharynx, oesophagus, crop (Orthoptera) or oesophageal diverticula (Nematocera : Muscidae) and a narrow valve like proventriculus or gizzard (Orthoptera).

Mesenteron is flask shaped and follows the proventriculus of the midgut. Its anterior narrow part is called cardia and the posterior relatively expanded part, the ventriculus or stomach proper.

At the junction of the midgut and hindgut are found Malpighian tubules that are blind tubes, bathed in blood and excretory in function.

Proctodaeum or the hindgut consists of ileum, colon, rectum and anus. Its internal anatomy is similar to the foregut.

2. CLASSIFICATION

The morphological bases of classification are chaetotaxy, wing-venation, mouthparts, genitalia, metamorphosis and certain special characters. In some instances, even bionomics and behavioural features also count. Phylum Arthropoda is divided into six classes:

CLASS : INSECTA

They have distinct head, thorax and abdomen; one pair of antennae and typically two pairs of wings on the 3-segmented thorax. Abdomen consists of ten segments of which the terminal one is modified for sexual purposes. Respiration is tracheate and various types of metamorphoses are met with.

SUBCLASS : PTERYGOTA

May be winged or secondarily wingless.

SERIES : EXOPTERYGOTA

ORDER : BLATTARIA

Dorso-ventrally flattened with smooth, tough integument; two pairs of wings in most species; head flexed downward and backward when at rest; antennae filiform and many segmented. Mouthparts are adapted for biting and chewing. Example : Cockroaches.

ORDER : ORTHOPTERA

Medium to large sized; have chewing, mandibulate mouth parts; wings present or absent; females generally with well-developed ovipositor which is concealed by the 7th or 8th abdominal sterna. Cerci are usually short and unsegmented. Example: Grasshoppers, locusts, crickets.

ORDER : HEMIPTERA

The order has been divided into 2 suborders : Heteroptera and Homoptera. In suborder Heteroptera, the base of rostrum does not touch anterior coxae; pronotum is large; forewings usually thickened basally and membranous apically, hind wings membranous, both pairs folded flat over the back with apices overlapping. Example : Bugs.

ORDER : ODONATA

Biting mouthparts; antennae very short and filiform; eyes large and prominent; abdomen elongate and slender; wings well developed with a complex reticulation of small cross-veins. Example : Dragonflies.

ORDER : MALLOPHAGA

Wingless with body compressed dorso-ventrally; tarsi are one or two clawed; mouthparts adapted for chewing. Example: Biting lice.

ORDER : ANOPLURA

Wingless with body compressed dorso-ventrally; tarsi are one-clawed, apposed by a toothed projection of the tibia; mouth parts adapted for piercing and sucking. Example : Sucking lice.

SERIES : ENDOPTERYGOTA

ORDER : COLEOPTERA

Minute to large-sized, hard-bodied insects; antennae 10-14 segmented; forewings modified into elytra which completely cover the abdomen, almost always meet to form a straight mid-dorsal line; hind wings membranous, folded underneath elytra or reduced or even wanting. Example : Beetles.

ORDER : HYMENOPTERA

Typically with 2 pairs of membranous unequal wings; hind wings smaller than forewings and the two are often interlocked. Some species have vestigial wings or wingless. Mouthparts are adapted for chewing and lapping; a narrow isthmus joins the thorax with the abdomen; compound eyes conspicuous; abdomen of female usually provided caudally with a "sting". Example : Bees, wasps, ants.

ORDER : LEPIDOPTERA

Have 2 pairs of membranous wings that are covered with overlapping scales; mouthparts coiled and adapted for sucking; no cerci. Example : Moths and butterflies.

ORDER : DIPTERA

With 1 pair of membranous wings attached to the second thoracic segment; second pair of wings modified into minute, club-shaped balancers or halters; mouth parts adapted for sucking. Example : Flies.

ORDER : SIPHONAPTERA

Wingless, with body strongly compressed laterally; have an especially long pair of hind legs, adapted for jumping; mouthparts are adapted for piercing and sucking. Example : Fleas.

CLASS : CRUSTACEA

Exoskeleton is thin and transparently membranous or thick and impregnated with calcium carbonate. Major divisions of the body are cephalon with five fused somites, paired antennules, antennae, mandibles, first thoracopod typically biramous with exopod and inner endopod arising from basal protopod.

ORDER : CYCLOPODA

Carapace absent; antennules are uniramous, more developed in male than in female; antennae uniramous, exopod absent or reduced; mandibles with biramous palpi. Example : *Cyclops*.

ORDER : DECAPODA

Carapace subcylindrical or ovoid; antennules are biramous; antennae with 5 segments; mandibles with palpi; maxillipedes with first endopod of 2 or fewer segments; thoracopod with uniramous appendages; telson appears like tail fan. Example : Crayfish and crab.

CLASS : DIPLOPODA

Have 2 pairs of legs and 2 pairs of spiracles per segment for the most part of body. Example : Millipede.

CLASS : CHILOPODA

Forms usually with a single pair of legs and 1 pair of spiracles for each of the post-cephalic segments of the body; first pair of legs modified to form poison claws. Example : Centipede.

CLASS : ARACHNIDA

Forms with body divided into cephalo-thorax and abdomen; without antennae; adults with 4 pairs of legs; chelicerae replace the sensory antennae.

ORDER : SCORPIONES

Body elongate; cephalo-thorax unsegmented; anterior part of abdomen is as broad as cephalo-thorax, composed of 7 segments; posterior abdomen narrowed with 6 flexible segments, of which the terminal one is differentiated into a pyriform poison organ ending in a hollow stinger spine. Example : Scorpions.

ORDER : ARANEAE

Cephalo-thorax distinctly constricted from the abdomen that is usually unsegmented; first pair of appendages (chelicerae) is 2-jointed with opening of poison gland through hollow fanged tip. Example : Spiders.

ORDER : ACARI

Cephalo-thorax and abdomen united, not externally segmented; adults with 4 pairs of legs, larvae with 3 pairs of legs. Example : Ticks and mites.

CLASS : PENTASTOMIDA

Elongate, tongue-like, cylindrical or moniliform, with many pseudo-segments, but no separation into head, thorax and abdomen; head with median subterminal mouth and 2 pairs of hollow retractile claws; eyes lacking; sexes separate, male smaller than female. Example : *Linguatula serrata* (tongue worm).

CLASS : INSECTA

Forms with distinct head, thorax and abdomen; with I pair of antennae; typically with 2 pairs of wings on the thorax which consists of 3 segments; have three pair of legs; abdomen composed of 10 segments of which the terminal one is modified for sexual purposes; respiration is tracheate; opening of the genital organs is near the caudal end of the body.

SUBCLASS : SYNAPTERA

They are wingless, primitive insects/descendants of wingless insects; ametabola; have one or more abdominal appendages; may have genitalia and cerci. Only the order Thysanura has veterinary/medical importance. Example : Silverfish, firebrats etc. that cause damage to books and cloths.

SUBCLASS : PTERYGOTA

Winged and wingless insects, descended from winged ancestors. This group includes many orders of insects, which are of medical/veterinary importance.

Class : Crustacea

Subclass : Copepoda

Order : Cyclopoda

Genus : *Cyclops*

(Plate : II)

Common name : Water flea. **Habitat** : Free-living in stagnant water, ponds, lakes and step-wells (Limnetic forms), some species occur in salt water (Littoral forms). **Distribution** : Cosmopolitan.

Size and Colour : Littoral forms are smaller than limnetic forms; the commonly occurring limnetic forms are usually colourless, semi-transparent, long and slender, with long caudal rami. In general, they are just visible to the naked eye and are without carapace but have a cephalic shield anteriorly. **Body** : Well segmented, possesses swimming feet at the thorax. Metastome (Cephalothorax) is wider than urostome (posterior part of the thorax) and ends in a median forked rostrum. **Antennae** : Two pairs, lying on either side of the anterior end of metastome. First pair of antennae is long, powerful, uniramous and 17 segmented. The second pair lies behind the first pair, is short, 4 segmented, biramous and powerful. **Abdomen** : Has 5 distinct segments, but has no appendages except caudal ramous at the extremity which possesses two limbs beset with bristles. **Eggs** : Are carried in sub-cylindrical sacs attached to the first abdominal segment on each side in females.

Economic importance : They act as vectors of *Diphyllobothrium latum*, *Dracunculus medinensis* and *Gnathosoma* spp.

Order : Decapoda

Genus : *Potamobius* (=*Astacus*)

(Plate : II)

Common name : Cray fish. **Habitat** : Marine, brackish or fresh water. **Distribution** : Worldwide except Africa and parts of Asia.

Body : Fish like, consists of 19 segments, anterior portion is known as cephalo-thorax and the posterior abdomen. The portion of carapace separating head from thorax is known as cervical groove or suture. **Head** : Bears a rostrum, compound eyes and two pairs of antennae. **Legs** : Many pairs, the first pair is modified into heavy pincers, the chelipeds. **Abdomen**: Has 6-7 segments and the last segment has broad, flat uropods, used for swimming.

Economic importance : Acts as vector of lungflukes (*Paragonimus* spp.).

Class : Chilopoda

Genus : *Scolopendra*

(Plate : II)

Common name : Common Indian centipede.

Size : Usually 10-15 cm. **Body** : Has head (red) and trunk (dirty yellow) and is elongate, segmented, dorso-ventrally flattened. **Head** : Bears a pair of filiform, jointed antennae; a pair of mandibles and two pairs of maxillae. **Trunk** : Has 21 segments, each having one lateral pair of 7-jointed legs. The legs end in claws. The appendages of first segment of trunk are strongly prehensile and bear poison fangs on their distal part.

Economic importance : Chiefly carnivorous, sometimes, during search of their shelters may enter the natural openings of vertebrates and produce considerable irritation.

Class : Diplopoda

Genus : *Thyroglutus*

(Plate : II)

Common name : Large tropical millipede. **Distribution** : Common in India. **Body** : Long, cylindrical and segmented. **Head** : Bears a pair of short-clubbed antennae, a pair of eyes, a pair of mandibles and a pair of maxillae. **Thorax** : Short and 4 segmented. **Abdomen** : Multi-segmented, each segment has two pairs of legs on either side. All the legs arise very close to the mid-ventral line.

Economic importance : Some millipedes possess a series of scent glands that secrete an irritating substance.

Class : Pentastomida

Order : Porcephalida

Family : Linguatulidae

Genus : *Linguatula*

Linguatula serrata

(Plate : II)

Common Name : Tongue worm

Hosts : Dogs, fox, wolf, rarely man, horse, sheep and goat. **Location** : Adults are found attached to nasal mucosa, occasionally pharynx, larynx and oesophagus by two pairs of hooks. **Distribution** : Cosmopolitan.

Size : Males smaller i.e. 1.8-2.0 cm. and females, 3-13 cm.

Body : Elongate, tongue shaped, convex dorsally, flattened ventrally and has transversely striated cuticle giving the appearance of pseudo-segments. **Mouth** : Sub terminal at the anterior end and surrounded by a chitinous ring. They have two pairs of hooks, one pair on either side of the mouth and the other behind. The hooks are situated on finger like projections and are retractile.

Economic importance : Causes respiratory disturbances like sneezing, coughing, dyspnoea in its hosts.

Class : Insecta

Subclass : Pterygota

Order : Blattaria

Family : Blattidae

Periplaneta americana

(Plate : III)

Common name : American cockroach. **Distribution** : Cosmopolitan, very common in India.

Size : 28-44 mm. **Colour** : Chestnut brown. **Wings** : Extend beyond the tip in males and just cover the tip in females. **Thorax** : Has pale yellow area around the edge of pronotum. **Cercus** : the last segment is twice as long as wide.

Economic importance : May act as intermediate host for *Gongylonema neoplasticum* and *Hymenolepis diminuta* of rodents. Can mechanically transmit a number of viruses, bacteria, fungi, helminths and protozoa in human beings.

Class : Insecta

Order : Orthoptera

(Plate : III)

Examples : Grasshoppers, locusts. **Distribution** : More abundant in tropics than in temperate zones.

The representatives differ from the cockroaches in having well developed hind femur modified for jumping with coxae wide apart.

A few members such as *Melanoplus* and *Chrotogonus* (locusts), *Conocephalus* (grasshoppers) act as intermediate hosts of helminths.

Order : Odonata

(Plate : III)

Example : Dragonfly. **Distribution** : Neotropical and oriental regions.

They have long bodies, two pairs of delicate wings and strong capability for flight.

Economic importance : Their naiads (nymphs) carry the cercariae of the oviduct fluke, *Prosthogonimus* of ducks and fowls.

Class : Insecta

Order : Coleoptera

(Plate : III)

Example : Beetles.

Body : Integument is leathery and horny. **Mouthparts** : Chewing type. **Wings** : Two pairs. Forewings are called elytra, are hard, horny and act as covers. Hind wings are membranous and are used in flight. At rest, the elytra characteristically meet along a straight mid-dorsal line. **Larvae** : Are called grubs and usually have three pairs of well-developed legs.

Economic importance : Some genera of beetles such as *Anthicus, Dermestes, Gonocephalum, Sphenariopsis, Tenebrio* and *Tribolium* act as intermediate hosts of helminths.

Order : Hymenoptera

(Plate : III)

Examples : Ants, bees, wasps.

Mouthparts : Chewing or lapping type. **Wings** : Two pairs of membranous wings with few veins. The hind wings are smaller than the forewings. **Thorax and abdomen** : A well-marked constriction called isthmus is seen at the junction of thorax and abdomen. Abdomen of female often possesses a sting at the ovipositor. **Pupae** : Exarate type.

Economic importance : A few genera of ants act as intermediate hosts of helminths e.g. *Tetramorium* and *Pheidole* for *Raillietina (R.) tetragona, Monomorium* for *Cotugnia digonopora* and *Formica* for *Dicrocoelium dendriticum*.

Order : Hemiptera

Suborder : Heteroptera

Family : Cimicidae

Genus : *Cimex*

***Cimex hemipterus* (=*C. rotundatus*)**

(Plate : IV)

Common name : Bed bugs.

Hosts : Man, chicken etc. **Distribution** : Tropical and subtropical regions including India.

Size : 4-5 mm long. **Colour** : Dark brown. **Body** : Flat, elongate or ovoid in shape and is covered with characteristic spinose bristles. **Head** : Small, narrow and somewhat rounded. The compound eyes project conspicuously at the sides of the head. Ocelli are absent. **Antennae** : Long and four segmented. First segment is very short. **Mouthparts** : Piercing and sucking type. Mandibles penetrate and maxillae form a tube. Labium is three segmented. **Wings** : Vestigial. Forewings in adults are represented by two small brown pads on the dorsal surface of thorax. **Thorax** : The prothorax is large and notched anteriorly, where the head is inserted in it. The sides of pronotum are rounded. Stink glands are present in the last segment in adults. **Abdomen** : Has eight visible segments. Spiracles are located in segments 2 to 8 laterally. **Eggs** : Creamy white, 1 mm long and are with operculum.

Economic importance : In heavy infestation, they may cause severe irritation and anaemia in birds as well as in children.

C. lectularius

(Plate : IV)

Distribution : Temperate and subtropical regions; does not occur in India.

It differs from *C. hemipterus* in having less dark colour, wider and longer head, deeply notched pronotum with width 3 times the length at its middle, and a more rounded abdomen.

Economic importance : Same as of *C. hemipterus*.

Class : Insecta

Order : Mallophaga (Biting lice)

Suborder : Amblycera

Antennae : 4-5 segmented, lie in grooves. **Maxillary palps** :

Visible and are 2-5 segmented. **Thorax** : Meso- and meta-thorax fused and indistinct. **Abdomen** : With 8-10 visible segments. Most of them affect birds, except *Heterodoxus* spp.

Family : Menoponidae

Head : Broadly triangular, strongly enlarged at temples.

Menopon gallinae

(Plate : V)

Common name : Shaft louse of poultry. **Hosts** : Poultry including chicken, duck, pigeon, turkey and guinea fowl. **Distribution** : Probably worldwide.

Size : Male 1.71 mm; female 2.04 mm in length. **Colour** : Pale yellow. **Body** : On each thoracic and abdominal segment, there is one row of bristles. **Eyes** : Lodged in shallow pits. **Tarsi** : End in two claws. **Eggs** : Laid singly on feathers of breast and thigh region.

Economic importance : Due to irritation, there are production losses.

Menacanthus (=*Eomenacanthus*) *stramineus*

(Plate : V)

Common name : Large body louse of poultry. **Hosts** : Fowl, duck, turkey, pheasants and peacock. **Location** : Occurs on less feathered parts like breast, thigh, vent, etc. **Distribution** : Widespread in the world, more common in temperate zones including the hilly areas of India.

Size : Male 2.8 mm; female 3.3 mm in length. **Colour** : Yellow. **Head** : With ventral spine-like processes arising latero-posterior to the mandibles. **Abdomen** : The segments have alternate rows of large and small sized bristles. **Eggs** : Laid in clusters on feathers near the skin.

Economic importance : Same as of *M. gallinae*.

Suborder : Ischnocera

Antennae : Filiform, 2-5 segmented and are visible at the sides of the head. **Maxillary palps** : Absent. **Thorax** : Meso- and meta-thorax distinct. They are parasites on birds and mammals.

Family : Philopteridae

Pronotum : Strongly developed. **Antennae** : 5-segmented in both sexes. **Tarsi** : Bear 2 claws. They occur exclusively on birds.

Columbicola columbae

(Plate : V)

Common name : Pigeon louse. **Hosts** : Pigeons and doves. **Distribution** : Cosmopolitan.

Size : 2 mm in length. **Body** : Long, slender, elongated in front of the antennae. **Abdomen** : Has series of brown coloured areas corresponding with segments.

Economic importance : Heavy infestation causes loss of condition in pigeons.

Lipeurus caponis

(Plate : V)

Common name : Wing louse of poultry and pheasants. **Distribution** : Cosmopolitan.

Size : 2 mm in length. **Colour** : Very light. **Head** : Longer than its width but well rounded in front. There is post-antennal constriction in the male. **Antennae** : First antennal segment of male with dorsal appendage. **Body** : Narrow. There is one patch of long setae on each postero-lateral angle of metathorax.

Abdominal segments have transverse median sclerites.

Economic importance : Heavy infestation causes restlessness in birds.

Goniocotes gallinae

(Plate : V)

Common name : Fluff louse of poultry. **Hosts** : Fowl, pheasant and pigeon. **Location** : Basal parts of large feathers.

Size : Very small, 0.75-1.00 x 0.40 mm. **Shape** : Almost globular in outline. **Head** : Broader than long, has two long setae on each side in the post antennal region. **Antennae** : Are filiform and do not show sexual dimorphism.

Economic importance : Heavy infestation causes production losses.

Goniodes gigas

(Plate : VI)

Common name : Large chicken louse. **Host** : Fowl. **Distribution** : More common in tropics.

Size : 2-3 mm, often up to 5.0 mm. Are much bigger than *Goniocotes*. **Colour**: Head, thorax and legs are yellowish with dark markings. **Head** : Wider than long, has rounded front and angulate temples. There are more than 2 setae on each side of head in the post-antennal region. **Antennae** : Show no sexual dimorphism and are filiform.

Economic importance : Same as of *Goniocotes gallinae*.

Family : Trichodectidae

Antennae : 3-5 segmented. **Pronotum** : Strongly developed. **Abdomen** : Consists of more than 7 segments. **Tarsi** : End in a single claw.

Trichodectes canis
(Plate : VI)

Common name : Dog louse. **Hosts** : Dogs, also cats, jackals and other wild canines. **Location** : Base of hairs of head, neck and tail region. **Distribution** : Cosmopolitan.

Size : Short and broad. Males are 1.7 mm and females 1.9 mm in length. **Head** : Sub-quadrangular, the width is greater than length. **Colour** : Yellowish with dark markings. **Antennae** : Show sexual dimorphism. The first segment of antennae of male is enlarged.

Economic importance : Acts as vector of tapeworm (*Dipylidium caninum*) of dogs.

Family : Linognathidae

Most of them are parasitic on ungulates. **Head** : Longer than its width. **Eyes** : Absent. **Spiracles** : In six pairs. **Paratergal plates** : Absent. **Legs** : Progressively bigger from first to third pair. **Abdomen** : Membranous with hairs on the segments.

Linognathus vituli
(Plate : VI)

Common name : Long nosed cattle louse. **Location** : Dewlap, shoulders, sides of neck and rump. In heavy infestations the entire body may be covered. **Distribution** : Cosmopolitan, common in India.

Size : 2.0-2.5 mm in length. **Head** : Much longer than broad. **Abdomen**: Clothed with short setae, abdominal tergites with 2 rows of bristles. Pleural angles have 2 bristles each. **Paratergal plates** : Absent.

Economic importance : They cause louse worry, which is

characterized by licking, scratching and rubbing. As the coat becomes rough, secondary infections may occur. Heavy infestations may lead to anaemia.

Family : Haematopinidae

Head : Is without eyes but with ocular points and is deeply inserted into the thorax, forming temporal angles behind the antennae. **Thorax** : Sternal plates well developed. **Abdomen**: Paratergal plates also well developed and appear as sclerotized caps. **Legs** : Equal in size.

Haematopinus eurysternus

(Plate : VI)

Common name : Short nosed cattle louse. **Location** : Head and neck, tips of ears, base of tail. **Distribution** : Cosmopolitan.

Size : 3.5 – 4.7 mm. Longer and broader than *Linognathus vituli*. **Head** : Slightly longer than its width.

Economic importance : Same as in case of *L. vituli.*

H. suis

(Plate : VI)

Common name : Large sucking louse of hogs. **Location** : Folds of skin behind the ears and between the legs. **Distribution** : Cosmopolitan. It is the only louse affecting pigs.

Size : Largest species affecting livestock, 6-7 mm long. **Thoracic sternal plates** : Wider than long. **Paratergal plates** : Rounded.

Economic importance : It causes irritation, restlessness etc.

H. tuberculatus

(Plate : VI)

Common name : Large sucking louse of buffalo. **Location** : Chiefly on ears but may spread all over the body.

Distribution : Asia, Australia and Africa. **Hosts** : Buffalo, cattle, camel and yak. .

Size : Up to 5.5 mm. **Head** : Length and width subequal. **Abdomen** : Para-tergal plates prominent, pleural angles with 5 or more bristles.

Economic importance : Same as of *L. vituli.*

Order : Siphonaptera (Fleas)

(Plate : VII)

Body : Wingless, laterally compressed, somewhat pointed anteriorly, 1.5 to 4.0 mm in size. **Exoskeleton** : Thick and dark brown. **Eyes** : Compound eyes are absent; some species may have simple eyes. **Antennae** : Club- shaped, 3-jointed, lodged in grooves. **Thorax** : Usually smaller than head, possesses 3-pairs of legs. **Abdomen** : Has ten segments. The 9th segment is covered by sensory setae called sensilium or pygidium. **Comb/ctenidia** : Some fleas have a number of backwardly directed and powerful spines on cheeks or gena, known as genal comb/genal ctenidium and on posterior border of 1st thoracic segment, known as pronotal comb/pronotal ctenidium. **Legs** : Strong, long and adapted for leaping.

Family : Pulicidae

Head : Evenly rounded along margin. **Abdomen** : Tergites possess single row of setae.

Pulex irritans

(Plate : VII)

Common name : Human flea. **Hosts** : Mainly human beings may attack horses, dogs, calves, hogs and rodents. **Distribution** : Cosmopolitan.

Head : Frons are smoothly rounded, genal comb is absent. Ocular bristle is present below the eye. **Thorax** : Pronotal comb is absent. Mesosternite is not divided by a distinct vertical rod like sclerotization. **Abdomen** : The antipygidial bristles are short.

Economic importance : Sucks blood and may cause dermatitis and pruritus. May act as vector of *Dirofilaria immitis*.

Xenopsylla cheopis

(Plate : VII)

Common name : Human plague flea, Indian rat flea, oriental rat flea, tropical rat flea. **Hosts** : Rats are the natural hosts but the flea also attacks human beings, cats and other domestic animals. **Distribution** : Tropical and subtropical regions.

This flea resembles *P. irritans* except that (i) Ocular bristle is situated just in front of eye, (ii) Mesopleuron is wide and is divided by a distinct vertical rod like sclerotization and (iii) The antipygidial bristles are long.

Economic importance : It sucks blood from its hosts and is the chief vector of plague organisms, *Yersinia pestis*, responsible for bubonic plague in human beings. May also act as vector of murine typhus and of *Hymenolepis diminuta* and *H. nana*.

Ctenocephalides canis

(Plate : VII)

Common name : Dog flea. **Hosts** : Dogs, jackals, may attack other animals including man. **Distribution** : Cosmopolitan.

Head : Evenly rounded along the margins and about 1½ time as long as wide. Genal comb is having 7-8 spines and the first or frontal spine is shorter than the second spine. **Thorax** : Pronotal comb is present.

Economic importance : Sucks blood and acts as vector of tapeworm (*Dipylidium caninum*) and filarial worm (*Dipetalonema reconditum*).

C. felis

(Plate : VII)

Common name : Cat flea. **Hosts** : Cats, may attack other livestock animals. **Distribution** : Cosmopolitan.

This flea resembles *C. canis* except that (i) Head is longer than that of *C. canis* and (ii) Frontal/first spine of the genal comb is as long as the second spine.

Economic importance : Sucks blood of its hosts and may act as vector of *D. caninum*.

Family : Hectopsyllidae

The three thoracic tergites together are shorter in width than the first abdominal tergite.

Echidnophaga gallinacea

(Plate : VII)

Common name : Stick-tight flea of poultry. **Hosts** : Chickens and other birds. May attack horse, dog, cat, rabbit, rat and man.

Distribution : Tropical and sub-tropical countries including India.

Head : Frons is sharply angulated and the frontal margin of head is having two angles. **Thorax** : Dorsally narrower than the first abdominal segment. **Combs**: Both genal and pronotal combs are absent.

Economic importance : Causes progressive anaemia and emaciation in birds leading to reduce egg production in laying hens. In young birds there may be blindness and even death.

Order : Diptera

Includes mosquitoes, gnats and flies. There are three suborders, namely **Nematocera**, **Brachycera** and **Cyclorrhapha**.

Characters	Nematocera	Brachycera	Cyclorrhapha
Antennae	More than six jointed, mostly alike segments. Arista: Absent.	Less than six jointed, mostly non-alike segments. Arista: Absent in species of veterinary importance.	Three segmented. The distal segment has an outgrowth called arista.
Larvae	Have well developed head. Mandibles bite horizontally.	Have incomplete head. Mandibles bite vertically.	Have vestigial head; commonly called maggots.
Pupae	Obtectate	Obtectate	Coarctate
Habitat of developing stages	Aquatic	Aquatic	Terrestrial

Suborder : Nematocera
Family : Culicidae
(Plates : VIII to X)

Common name : Mosquitoes. **Body** : Slender with small, spherical head and long legs. **Antennae** : 14-16 segmented, show sexual dimorphism. **Proboscis**: Long and slender. **Thorax** : Wedge shaped. **Abdomen** : Elongated. **Wings** : Long, narrow, folded flat on abdomen while at rest; wing-veins covered with scalcs.

Salient morphological differences between Anophelinae and Culicinae are as follows :

Stage	Anophelinae	Culicinae
Eggs	Laid singly in water; provided with floats.	Laid in rafts (*Culex*) or singly (*Aedes*) in water, mud or places to be flooded with water.
Larvae	Lack respiratory siphon; possess pecton on VIII abdominal segment; palmate bristles present; float and rest parallel to the water surface; are surface feeders.	Possess respiratory siphon on VIII abdominal segment; lack palmate bristles; float and rest at an angle with the surface of water having the end of siphon applied to the surface. Feed slightly below the surface of water.
Pupae	Have short funnel shaped two respiratory trumpets; paddles at the tip of abdomen have an accessory hair in addition to a terminal hair.	Have breathing trumpets of various sizes e.g. long and slender in *Culex*; short and broad in *Aedes*; paddle tips with terminal hair only.
Head of adults	Palps of both male and female long; those of male clubbed and female non-clubbed.	Palps of male as long as or longer than proboscis, non-clubbed, those of female $1/5^{th}$ – ½ of the length of proboscis and non-clubbed.
Adults	Wings usually spotted or dappled; rest at an oblique angle with the surface	Wings usually unspotted or non-dappled; rest with body parallel to surface.

Economic importance : They suck blood and different species act as vectors of number of protozoan (*Plasmodium vivax, P. falciparum, P. gallinaceum* etc.), helminths (*Wuchereria bancrofti*, *Brugia malayi*, *Dirofilaria immitis*), viral (Japanese B encephalitis, yellow fever, Dengue fever, fowl pox virus, Eastern and Western equine encephalitis) and rickettsial organisms (*Borrelia anserina*).

Family : Ceratopogonidae

Genus : *Culicoides*

(Plate : XI)

Common name : Biting midges, punkies, gnats, no-se-ums. **Hosts** : Warm blooded animals including man. **Distribution** : Cosmopolitan.

Size : Extremely small, 0.6-5.0 mm. **Body** : Dark in colour. **Mouthparts** : Piercing and sucking type, palps having 5 segments of which the 3rd segment is enlarged. **Antennae** : Long, 14-segmented with beaded appearance; plumose in males and pilose in females. **Thorax** : Humped over the head. **Wings** : Have no scales but hairs are present. Wings are superimposed at the back during rest. **Legs** : Short and stout.

Economic importance : Several species act as vectors of nematodes (*Dipetalonema*, *Onchocerca*) and viral infections (Blue tongue of sheep, Venezuelan equine encephalitis).

Family : Simuliidae

Genus : *Simulium*

(Plate : XI)

Common name : Black fly, buffalo gnat. **Hosts** : Domestic and wild mammals, birds and man. **Distribution** : Cosmopolitan.

Size : 1.5 –6.0 mm, short and stout insects. **Body** : Mostly black, may be yellow or orange in colour; covered with short, golden and silvery hairs. **Antennae** : Long, 11-segmented and bare; do not show sexual dimorphism. **Eyes** : Holoptic in males and dichoptic in females. **Thorax** : Arched and is humped over the head. **Wings** : Broad, non- spotted, have no scales or hairs. The anterior wing veins are thickened while the other veins are faintly seen. **Legs** : Short and stout.

Economic importance : They act as vectors of a number of protozoan (*Leucocytozoon smithi*, *L simondi*), viral (Eastern equine encephalitis) and nematodes (*Onchocerca gutturosa*, *O. volvulus* etc.).

Family : Psychodidae

Genus : *Phlebotomus*

(Plate : XI)

Common name : Sand flies, owl midges, moth flies. **Hosts** : Man, dog and other domestic animals. **Distribution** : Mainly tropical and sub-tropical regions.

Size : Minute flies, measuring 2-4 mm in size. **Body** : Dull-grayish in colour, covered with long, coarse hairs. **Antennae** : Long, 16-segmented with beaded appearance. They are plumose in males and pilose in females. **Wings** : Hairy, held upward and outward at an angle of 60^0 with the body at the time of rest. Wing-veins are more or less parallel; there are no cross-veins except at the base. **Legs** : Long.

Economic importance : Acts as vector of visceral (*Leishmania donovani*, *L infantum*) and cutaneous leishmanosis (*L. tropica*, *L. brasiliensis*) as well as of rickettsial (*Bartonella bacilliformis*) and viral diseases (sand fly fever, vesicular stomatitis etc.).

Suborder : Brachycera

Family : Tabanidae

Size : Large sized flies, 5-25 mm in length. **Mouthparts** : Piercing and sucking type. **Antennae** : Short, 3-segmented and terminate in annulations. **Wings**: With well developed wing-veins and a characteristic discal cell.

Genus : *Tabanus*

(Plates : XII & XIII)

Common name : Horse fly, hippo fly, elephant fly, marsh fly, gad fly, breeze fly etc. **Hosts** : Horse, mule, cattle, buffalo, camel and sometimes man. **Distribution** : Cosmopolitan.

Size : Medium to large sized, may be up to 30 mm long. **Body** : Dull grayish in colour and almost bristle-less. **Eyes** : Large and prominent. **Antennae** : Three segmented, first segment is short and the 3rd segment is large with a tooth like projection at its base and four annulations. **Mouthparts** : Short and blade like. On dorsal side is the labrum, which has epipharynx, having the shape of a double-edged sword. There is a pair of mandibles, which move like scissors. On either side beneath the mandibles lie two maxillae, which are long and slender and have teeth at their distal end. They bear prominent maxillary palps. Hypopharynx is long and slender and is having salivary duct. On ventral side is the labium, which is having two labella on the distal end. Labella are having numerous fine channels, known as pseudotracheae. **Wings** : Clear and the discal cell is hexagonal in shape. **Larva** : The mature larva is grayish white in colour, have three thoracic and nine abdominal segments in addition to head. The body is cylindrical and tapers at both the ends. Fleshy tubercles are present on segments 3-10. The last segment is provided with a tracheal siphon, used for breathing.

Economic importance : Their bites are painful and irritating. They act as mechanical vectors of surra (*Trypanosoma evansi*).

Genus : *Chrysops*

(Plates : XII & XIII)

Common name : Deer fly, mangrove fly. **Hosts** : Deer; simians and man though may attack other animals. **Distribution** : Cosmopolitan.

Size : Smaller than *Tabanus*. **Eyes** : Brilliantly coloured, chiefly green. **Antennae**: Long, 3-segmented, 1st and 2nd segments are large, 3rd segment has 4-annulations. **Proboscis** : Longer than that of *Tabanus* and *Haematopota*. **Wings** : With hexagonal discal cell and a dark transverse cross band. **Abdomen** : Ovoid with yellow bands and dark stripes.

Economic importance : These flies act as vectors of *Trypanosoma* spp., *Pasteurella tularensis* and nematode (*Loa loa*).

Genus : *Haematopota*

(Plates : XII & XIII)

Common name : Brim, clegs, stouts. **Hosts** : Mainly cattle, pig and man. **Distribution** : Cosmopolitan, abundant in Africa.

Size : Moderate. **Body** : Brown in colour. **Antennae** : 3-segmented, 1st segment is large and bulbous, 2nd segment is very narrow and 3rd segment has 3-annulations. **Wings**: Gray in colour with hexagonal discal cell. Wings are having scroll like markings or dense mottling. **Abdomen** : Slender. **Legs** : Hind tibia is without spur at the tip.

Economic importance : Acts as vector of *Trypanosoma theileri* in cattle.

Suborder : Cyclorrhapha

Series : Schizophora

Super family : Acalypterae

Mostly small sized, rarely exceed 3.0 mm in length. The 2nd antennal segment is without a longitudinal cleft on its upper outer edge. The transverse suture on thorax, between scutum and scutellum is incomplete.

Family : Gasterophilidae

Genus : *Gasterophilus*

Gasterophilus intestinalis

(Plate : XIV)

Common name : Horse bot fly. The larvae are known as stomach bots or horse bots. **Hosts** : Equines and also man. **Distribution** : Cosmopolitan.

Size : 11-15 mm. **Body** : Pale yellow to dark in colour, covered with hairs. **Mouthparts** : Vestigial and arista is bare. **Wings** : Transparent with dark spots which form an irregular dark transverse band across the centre of the wing. **Abdomen** : Yellowish brown in colour with its end bent forward under the body. **Legs** : The hind coxa in male shows a spatulate process and in female a tubercle is there. **Eggs** : Yellowish, cemented directly to the distal part of the hair and are without pedicel, pointed at the proximal part, operculated at the distal end and transversely striated. They appear as wedge shaped in lateral view and measure 1.25 mm in length. **Larva** : The mature or 3rd stage larvae are yellow or pink in colour, barrel shaped and measure up to 20 mm in length. There are two rows of spines, extending up to 10th segment and rarely up to 11th. The last 2-3 dorsal rows of spines are medially interrupted. The spines of first row are larger than that of second row. **Posterior spiracles** : Are present in a spiracular pouch which is semicircular having bow shaped slits.

Economic importance : Larval stages cause digestive disturbances in equines. Heavy infestations may cause death of the host.

Gasterophilus nasalis

(Plate : XIV)

Common name : Throat bot fly and the larvae are known as stomach bots or horse bots. **Hosts** : Equines and rarely man. **Distribution** : South America, Australia and India.

Size : 8-13 mm, smaller than *G. intestinalis*. **Wings** : Unspotted. **Eggs** : Yellowish, cylindrical with dome like operculum; have no pedicel. They remain attached to the proximal part of the hair and do not stand away from the hair. They are elongate to ovoid and 1.3 mm in length. **Larva** : The mature or 3rd stage larvae are 14 mm in size, have one row of spines on segments 3-11, and denticles up to 11th segment. The spines on the ventral side of the 3rd row may be missing. **Posterior spiracles** : Morphologically resemble with those of *G. intestinalis*.

Economic importance : The larval stages cause respiratory and digestive disturbances in equines.

Genus : *Cobboldia*

Cobboldia elephantis

(Plate : XIV)

Common name : Elephant bot fly. **Hosts** : Elephants. **Distribution** : India, Sri Lanka and Myanmar.

Size : 15-20 mm. **Body** : Flattened. **Mouthparts** : Vestigial. **Head** : The frons is strongly protruding; in females it is as broad as length of the eye and in males it is distinctly narrower. Head is predominantly bright orange in colour. **Thorax, abdomen and legs** : Shiny black in colour. **Eggs** : 1.8-1.9 mm long, yellowish in colour. **Larva** : Mature/3rd stage larvae are 10-28 mm in length and have single, large, pointed mouth hook. Mouth is surrounded by a crown of teeth, which are long and sharp on ventral side. The segments 8-9 bear 2-6 rows of spines dorsally; ventrally these spines may be up to the 12th segment. **Posterior spiracles** : Bear three pairs of straight slits, are completely eclipsed by the last segment.

Economic importance : Larval stages cause digestive disturbances.

Superfamily : Calypterae

Family : Oestridae

Genus : *Oestrus*

Oestrus ovis

(Plate : XV)

Common name : Sheep nasal bot fly. **Hosts** : Sheep, goat and occasionally camel. **Distribution** : Cosmopolitan, very common in India.

Size : 8-15 mm. **Body** : Has far less and relatively short bristles compared to other bot flies. **Head** : Yellow to light brown with prominent pock-like pits localized in between the eyes and below them. **Antennae** : Arista is bare. **Mouthparts** : Vestigial. **Wings** : Hyaline and have fourth longitudinal vein curved forward at the tip. **Larva** : The mature/3rd stage larva is 20.0 – 30.0 mm long, yellow when young, changing to a light brown later and shows broad transverse blackish bands dorsally. The segments bear 2-5 rows of strong spines ventrally, which are irregularly placed on the third segment but are fairly regular on the following segments. **Posterior spiracles** : D-shaped with a central button and without a distinct suture. Spiracular openings are arranged in a radiating fashion. **Pupa** : Coarctate, black, weakly wrinkled, 15-16 mm long, generally found in soil.

Economic importance : The larval stages cause respiratory and sometimes nervous disorders in sheep.

Genus : *Cephalopina*

Cephalopina titillator

(Plate : XV)

Common name : Camel nasal bot fly. **Host** : Camel. **Distribution** : Wherever camels are found.

Head : With orange upper and pale yellow lower parts. **Eyes** : Dichoptic in female and holoptic in male. **Thorax** : Dark brown to black. **Wings** : Transparent, the upper marginal cross veins are strongly sigmoid. **Abdomen** : With irregular spotted pattern. **Larva** : Mature/3rd stage larva measures up to 32.0 mm, has rows of smooth fleshy processes on segments 3 – 9. **Posterior spiracles** : Situated in deep furrows, consist of 2 large, black, kidney shaped borders with convergent rows of openings. The spiracular plates are placed obliquely with their anterior end near the median line. The spiracular buttons are located on the extreme median side. **Pupa** : 17.0 x 7.0 mm, strongly convex dorsally and shows direct conspicuous fleshy processes.

Economic importance : Larval stages cause respiratory disorders.

Genus : *Hypoderma*

Hypoderma lineatum

(Plate : XV)

Common name : Ox warble fly or heel fly. **Hosts** : Cattle. **Distribution** : More common in Canada and USA, but widely distributed in other regions including India.

Size : Usually 12.0-13.0 mm in length, may be up to 17.0 mm when the ovipositor is extended. **Body** : Black with bands of varying shades of yellow or orange hairs. **Mouthparts** : Proboscis is vestigial and inserted in a deep slit. **Antennae** : Arista is bare. **Wings** : Slightly smoky; may be dark brown or black; fourth longitudinal wing vein curves forward at the tip. **Thorax** : Yellow, except at the dorsum, which has black and white hairs; four longitudinal shiny black lines are present on the dorsal surface. **Eggs** : Elongate, pale yellow with smooth shiny surface, ovoid and attached to the proximal part of the hair at an angle of 45^0. As many as 20 eggs may be attached in a row by means of a clasp and a stalk. **Larva** : 3rd stage larva varies from yellow, yellow brown to dark brown in colour as it matures. It is barrel shaped, concave dorsally and convex ventrally, relatively more tapering at the anterior end. The spines are present ventrally from segments 2 - 10. It completely lacks hooks or cephalopharyngeal skeleton, has tubercles on ventral surface. **Posterior spiracles** : Kidney shaped, slightly depressed in the centre with radiating furrows of annulations. The posterior stigmal plates are flat and space in between the plates is relatively wider. **Pupa** : Coarctate. The character of stigmal plates of 3rd stage larva is maintained and is helpful in identification. Colour changes from brown to black while completing pupation.

Economic importance : The larval stages cause downgrading of carcass at slaughter and holes made by the larvae decrease the value of the hide. The flies cause gadding in cattle.

Hypoderma bovis

(Plate : XV)

Hosts : Cattle. **Distribution** : More common in Europe but found in India also.

Size : Adult 15 mm, stouter of the two ox warble flies. The bands on body measure more than 5.0 mm in width. **Thorax** : Broader and hairless; longitudinal lines on the dorsum are far less distinct. **Wings** : Wing veins are dark brown. **Eggs** : Laid singly and are slightly bigger. **Larva** : Comparatively bigger. The 3rd stage larva has rows of spines and tubercles ventrally on segments 2 - 9.

Economic importance : Larval stages cause formation of jelly like tracks in muscles. The breathing holes made by the larvae decrease value of the hide, which is used as leather.

H. crossi

Hosts : Goat and sheep, rarely cattle. **Distribution** : Found in the Indian subcontinent only.

Size : 11.5-12.0 mm. **Thorax** : Has distinct narrow black stripes on dorsum. **Wings** : Have numerous rills on the posterior border. **Eggs** : Laid in a row like *H. lineatum* but they are not provided with stalk between the body of the egg and clasp. **Larva** : The mature larva bears rows of spines and tubercles on segments 2–8, ventrally. **Posterior spiracles** : Appear excavated and have radiating furrows.

Economic importance : Larval stages cause depreciation in the value of carcass and hide.

H. diana

Common name : Deer warble fly. **Hosts** : Deer : **Distribution** : Wide, Western Europe across Central Asia to Far East. Occurs in India also.

Size : Adults identical to *H. lineatum*. **Wings** : Hyaline with yellow veins. **Eggs** : Similar to those of *H. lineatum*. **Larva** : Mature larva measures up to 25 mm in length.

Economic importance : Heavy infestation may cause severe ill health or death of deer.

Family : Muscidae

Genus : *Musca*

(Plate : XVI)

Common name : Housefly. **Hosts** : Domestic livestock, birds and man. **Distribution** : Cosmopolitan, *M. vicina* and *M. nebulo* are common in India.

Size : Medium sized i.e. 6-7 mm long and 13-15 mm across the wings. **Eyes** : Holoptic in males and dichoptic in females. **Antennae** : Brown in colour and possess arista, which is bilaterally plumose up to the tip. **Mouthparts** : Consist of black club-shaped maxillary palps, retractile proboscis; the labium is expanded distally into two labella. Labella have pseudotracheae. A short labrum epipharynx is also present. **Thorax** : Females have four longitudinal dark stripes, which are equally broad and extend to the posterior border of the scutum. In males, the thorax is completely black. **Wings** : Fourth longitudinal wing vein (M_{1+2}) curves sharply forward and the apical cell (R_5) is nearly closed. **Abdomen** : The grayish abdomen has various light and dark markings. **Eggs** : Pearly white, oblong, about 1 mm in length. The dorsal surface is concave with two curved rib-like thickenings, which run almost parallel to each other. **Larva** : The mature/3rd stage larva measures 12 mm; creamy white with spinulations. **Anterior spiracles** : Have 5-7 branches. **Posterior spiracles :** Have well developed peritremes. The spiracular plates are 'D' shaped having a button and three winding slits each. The slits are roughly 'M' shaped. **Pupa** : Coarctate. Pupal stage passes through dirty yellow, reddish brown, mahogany and dark colours in quick succession. It measures 8-9 mm and shows imprints of the 3rd stage larva in the form of lines indicative of segments. Posterior spiracles are represented by two flat, button-like prominences at the posterior extremity.

Economic importance : These flies are responsible for the mechanical transmission of viral (poliomyelitis), bacterial (typhoid, enteric fever, cholera, anthrax, tuberculosis, leprosy etc), protozoa (*Entamoeba*) and helminthic infections (*Enterobius, Ascaris* etc.). *Musca domestica* acts as intermediate host for helminthic infections (*Habronema* spp, *Raillietina* spp), *M. autumnalis* for eye worm (*Thelazia rhodesii*) and *M. conducens* for *Stephanofilaria assamensis*.

Genus : *Stomoxys*

Stomoxys calcitrans

(Plate : XVII)

Common name : Stable fly, biting horse fly. **Hosts** : Domestic animals and man. **Distribution** : Cosmopolitan.

Size : 6.0-8.0 mm in length. **Colour** : Dark robust. **Antennae** : Have arista, which is plumose on the dorsal side only. **Mouthparts** : Proboscis is long, slender, strongly sclerotized and shining black or gray in colour, with small labella. It projects like a bayonet at the anterior end of the fly. The labium bears two rows of prominent teeth on the retractile labellum. The slender palps are less than half as long as proboscis. **Thorax** :

Has four longitudinal dark stripes of which the lateral ones are narrow and do not reach up to the posterior border of the scutum. **Wings** : The 4th longitudinal wing vein (M_{1+2}) curves gently upward and not angled, so the apical cell (R_5) is widely open. When at rest, the wings are spread widely apart. **Abdomen** : Broader and shorter than that of housefly and has dark spots on either side at the 2nd and 3rd segments, the 1st and 4th segments are without spots. **Eggs** : Dirty white to yellow in colour and measure 1.3 x 0.3 mm in size. They are curved on one side, straight and grooved on the other side. **Larva** : Young larva is white translucent, footless maggot and measures 0.25 - 1.8 mm in length. It is tapering at the anterior end and rounded at the posterior end. The mature larva reaches a length of 20.0 mm. It has a cephalopharyngeal skeleton and mouth hooks like other larvae but the head is narrower than that of *Musca*. **Anterior spiracles** : Bear five papillae. **Posterior spiracles** : The spiracular plates are brown in colour, triangular in outline and are placed considerably apart. They are not conspicuously raised and each plate possesses three 'S' shaped slits with a button in the centre. **Pupa** : Barrel shaped and measures 5-7 mm in length. It can be recognized by its posterior spiracles, which resemble those of 3rd stage larvae.

Economic importance : Acts as mechanical vector of protozoan (*Trypanosoma evansi, T. gambiense, T. rhodesiense, T. vivax*), bacterial (Anthrax, brucellosis) and viral infections (Equine infectious anaemia, African horse sickness). Also acts as intermediate host for *Habronema majus* and *Hymenolepis carioca*.

Genus : *Haematobia* (= *Lyperosia*)

(Plate : XVIII)

H. irritans irritans is commonly known as horn fly, whereas ***H. irritans exigua*** as buffalo fly.

Hosts : Buffalo, cattle, horse and dog. **Distribution** : The first named is mostly found in temperate regions while the latter species is more common in the oriental region, including India.

Size : Half the size of house fly, measures 2.5 - 5.0 mm in length, and is one of the smallest muscids. **Antennae** : Have arista haired on the dorsal side only. **Mouth parts** : The labium is heavier than that of *Stomoxys* and the stout, yellow palpi are almost as long as the dark proboscis or sub-equal. **Wings** : Wing venation is similar to *Stomoxys*; while biting, the wings are spread but at the time of resting on the animal, the wings are folded closely. **Thorax** : Silver gray medially, dark laterally and has two well defined dark stripes. **Eggs** : Long, oval, creamy, grooved on the concave side, measure 1 mm x 0.3 mm in size. **Larva** : Freshly hatched larva is white, transparent; when fully grown, it measures up to 10 mm. **Posterior spiracles** : 'D' shaped, having sinuous slits and a median button. **Pupa** : Dark brown, barrel shaped and 3.5 - 4.0 mm in length.

Economic importance : *Haematobia exigua* acts as a mechanical vector of *Trypanosoma evansi* and intermediate host of *Habronema majus*, whereas, *H. irritans* acts as intermediate host of *Stephanofilaria stilesi* of cattle.

Family : Calliphoridae

The flies are commonly known as blowflies as their wing beats make a loud buzzing sound at the time of oviposition. Their larvae may be saprophagous or thrive upon living tissues of vertebrates and invertebrates.

Genus : *Calliphora*

(Plate : XVIII)

Common name : Blue bottle fly. **Hosts** : Mainly sheep but other domestic animals may also be affected. **Distribution** : India, Russia and New Zealand.

Size : 5-14 mm, larger than *Lucilia* and *Chrysomyia*. **Colour** : Metallic blue. **Mouthparts** : The proboscis is lapping or spongy type and resembles with that of *Musca,* except that it is fleshier. **Eyes** : Red in colour, holoptic in males and dichoptic in females. **Antennae** : Bilaterally plumose, do not bear bristle terminally. **Thorax and abdomen** : Show bluish metallic sheen or luster. **Wings** : M_2 wing-vein bends strongly forward but does not close the apical cell. **Legs** : Black or black brown in colour. **Eggs** : 1.7 mm long, white in colour and banana shaped. **Larva** : The mature or 3rd stage larva measures 19 mm in size, has accessory oral sclerites and complete spinose bands on segments 2 - 9. **Anterior spiracles** : Have 7-10 branches. **Posterior spiracles** : Have a close peritreme with an enclosed button in the ring and three slits which are straight, elongate and directed inward rather almost horizontally. **Pupa** : Coarctate, barrel shaped and enclosed in the skin of the mature larva which forms the puparium.

Economic importance : Larval stages cause myiasis and immense economic losses due to decreased value of fleece, reduced meat and milk production and death in extreme cases.

Genus : *Lucilia*

(Plate : XIX)

Common name : Green bottle fly. **Hosts** : Domestic animals especially sheep. **Distribution** : *Lucilia cuprina* is common throughout Indian plains.

Size : 5-11 mm, slightly smaller than *Calliphora*. **Colour** : Bright metallic green. **Body** : Less bristly than *Calliphora*. **Head** : Ocellar triangle large, reaching half way to the lunule in the female. Genae are bare. **Eyes** : Brownish red in colour, holoptic in males and dichoptic in females. **Antennae** : Bear an arista, which is bilaterally plumose. **Wings** : Squamae are bare. Whole of 3rd longitudinal wing vein (R_{4+5}) may be spiny. **Thorax and abdomen** : Bright metallic green without any pattern, sometimes more or less coppery in both sexes. Thorax is having a number of spiny bristles. **Eggs** : Pale yellow white, about 1 mm in length. **Larva** : The mature/3rd stage larva measures up to 16 mm, has girdle of spinules complete on segments 2 - 8 and 11. The segment 10 has 1- 2 rows of bristles dorsally but they are mostly interrupted on segments 9 - 10 and invariably on segment 12. **Anterior spiracles** : With 7-8 branches. **Posterior spiracles** : With complete ring, having 3-barrel shaped slits, which run parallel. There is no button. **Pupa** : Dark brown, oval and is indistinguishable from other species.

Economic importance : Same as that of *Calliphora*.

Genus : *Chrysomyia*

(Plate : XIX)

Common name : Screwworm fly. **Hosts** : Domestic animals and also man. **Distribution** : *Chrysomyia bezziana* is the commonest Indian blowfly.

Size : 5-12 mm. **Colour** : Bluish green. **Body** : Less bristly than *Lucilia*. **Head** : Males of *C. bezziana* are easily separable from other species as the facets on the upper part of the eye are not demarcable from the lower part. Face is orange yellow in colour. **Antennae** : Feathered up to the tip. **Wings** : Squamae are hairy. Stem vein ciliates posteriorly on the upper surface of the wing. **Thorax and abdomen** : Possess longitudinal stripes and transverse bands respectively but bristles are absent. They show bluish green metallic sheen. **Legs** : Black or partly dark brown. **Eggs** : Pearly white, 1.25 mm long, slightly convex ventrally and concave dorsally. **Larva** : The mature or 3rd stage larva measures 9 - 18 mm in length. The last segment is provided with a pair of ventral finger-like tubercles, which have a frontal ridge with denticles. There are transverse rows of short, stout, light brown black-tipped, posteriorly directed spines on its segments. **Anterior spiracles** : Have 4-6 branches. **Posterior spiracles** : Have incomplete peritreme and do not enclose button, which is mostly ill defined, or absent. All the spiracular slits slope downward and inward. **Pupa** : Dark red to brown in colour, measures 9 - 10 mm in length and has transverse rows of spines as in third larval stage.

Economic importance : Same as that of *Calliphora*.

Family : Sarcophagidae

Genus : *Sarcophaga*

(Plate : XX)

Common name : Flesh fly. **Hosts** : Domestic animals and occasionally man. **Distribution** : Cosmopolitan. *Sarcophaga ruficornis* and *S. haemorrhoidalis* are important in India.

Size : Medium to large, measuring 10-15 mm in length. **Body** : Slender. **Antennae** : Possess long arista, which is bilaterally plumose up to the middle with the remaining distal part bare. **Wings** : M_1 and M_2 wing veins are sharply bent forward, nearly closing the radius cell (R_5). **Thorax** : Mesonotum with three broad longitudinal stripes. **Abdomen** : Gray black with chessboard pattern, the markings being variable with incidence of light. **Larva** : The mature/3rd stage larva is densely spinulose. **Posterior spiracles** : Have incomplete peritreme, lack buttons; the stigmata are in pits and spiracular slits are more or less vertical. **Pupa** : Bigger in size than that of *Musca* and has spiracular indentations which are lacking in *Musca*.

Economic importance : These flies cause myiasis in a septic wound.

Genus : *Wohlfahrtia*

(Plate : XX)

Hosts : Domestic animals and even man but camel and sheep are its special victims. **Distribution** : Southern Russia, Northern United States, Southern Canada, North Africa, Southern Europe and India.

Body : Less slender than that of *Sarcophaga.* **Antennae** : Arista short and bare or with slight plumosity, which does not reach the tip. **Abdomen** : Gray with rounded spots which are fixed and do not change with the incidence of light.

Economic importance : The flies cause traumatic cutaneous myiasis.

Suborder : Cyclorrhapha

Series : Pupipara

They lay larvae, which pupate immediately. Their integument is leathery and the body is dorso-ventrally flattened. The legs end in strong claws. Antennae are one jointed and lie in pits. Abdomen is sac like.

Family : Hippoboscidae

Genus : *Hippobosca*

(Plate : XXI)

Common name : Forest fly. **Hosts** : Dog, cattle, buffalo, horse, camel and also man. **Distribution** : Cosmopolitan, occurs in India.

Size : 1.0 cm in length. **Colour** : Reddish brown spotted with pale yellow marks. **Body** : Dorso-ventrally flattened with leathery integument. **Eyes** : Ocelli absent, compound eyes large and prominent. **Antennae** : One jointed with a terminal arista (Style). **Mouthparts** : Proboscis is retractile, ensheathed by two short palps, provided with a strong set of teeth on either side of prostomum. Mouthparts are of biting, piercing and sucking type. **Wings** : Well developed, subtriangular, shorter than the total length of the body. Wing veins are crowded at the anterior margin, rilled like a partly opened fan. **Abdomen** : Without apparent segmentation and saculate. **Legs** : Provided with stout claws. **Larva** : Third stage larva when fully mature is white in colour and has black post-abdominal spiracles. It is covered with black warts, turns yellow and becomes shining black pupa. **Pupa** : Subglobular, measures 4.4 x 3.8 mm in size. It is convex dorsally, flattened ventrally, flattened or slightly depressed anteriorly and truncated posteriorly.

Economic importance : Heavily infested animals show emaciation, anaemia and general unthriftiness.

Genus : *Lipoptena*

Common name : Deer ked. **Hosts** : Deer, goats and may attack other animals and man. **Distribution** : India, Europe and North America.

Size : Smaller than the 'Sheep ked'. **Eyes** : Ocelli are present. **Wings** : Both sexes possess wings on emergence from pupae and are called volants. They lose their wings during maturing process and the stumps may be visible. The females lose their wings when they find their mates.

Economic importance : Same as of *Hippobosca* spp.

Genus : *Pseudolynchia*

***P. canariensis* (= *P. maura*)**

(Plate : XXI)

Common name : Louse fly of pigeon, pigeon fly. **Distribution** : Tropical and subtropical parts of Europe, America, Asia including India. **Hosts** : Pigeons, doves etc.

Size : 6 mm in length. **Colour** : Dark brown. **Body** : Resembles that of 'sheep ked' except that it possesses wings. **Wings** : Present and are lanceolate, rounded at the tip, longer than the total length of the body. **Legs** : Provided with accessory tooth at the basal plate of tarsal claws.

Economic importance : They act as vector of protozoan parasite of birds (*Haemoproteus* spp.).

Genus : *Melophagus*

M. ovinus

(Plate : XXI)

Common name : Sheep ked or sheep tick. **Hosts** : Sheep and goat. **Distribution** : More common in temperate zones. In India, it mainly confines to hilly areas.

Size : 5-7 mm in length. **Colour** : Reddish brown. **Body** : Leathery, dorso-ventrally flattened with stiff bristles all over the body. **Head** : Short, broad, sunken into the thorax and is not freely movable. **Eyes** : Small. **Antennae** : One jointed; located in pits at the forehead. **Mouthparts** : Piercing and sucking type with retractile proboscis. **Wings** : Vestigial. Halters are absent. **Thorax** : Brown in colour. **Abdomen** : Grayish brown, broad and saculate. **Legs** : Strong and provided with a pair of stout claws.

Economic importance : Large populations of sheep ked may result in wool staining by their faeces causing downgrading of the fleece. They also transmit *Trypanosoma melophagium* in sheep.

Class : Arachnida

This is the second largest class of arthropods, which includes ticks, mites, spiders, scorpions etc. The members differ from Insecta in lacking antennae, wings and compound eyes, and in possessing 4-pairs of legs in the adult and nymphal stages. The first pair of appendages is modified to form prehensile/ cutting **chelicerae** and second pair of appendages form **pedipalps**. Head with mouthparts is termed as **gnathosoma**. The segmentation of thc rest of the body is indistinct or absent. The parts of the body other than gnathosoma are variously labelled, that bearing the legs as **podosoma** and the part behind the legs as **opisthosoma**.

A glossary of some of the common terms is as follows **(Plates : XXII to XXIV)** :

Camerostome : The mouthparts in soft ticks are not visible from the dorsal side and lie in a groove on the ventral side, called camerostome.

Capitulum : The anterior movable part of the body bearing the mouthparts viz. pedipalps, hypostome and chelicerae.

Basis capitulum : It is the chitinous basal part of capitulum.

Hypostome : It is a spatulate structure, medio-ventral and toothed with longitudinal rows of recurved teeth.

Chelicerae : Paired structures located dorso-lateral to the hypostome and provided with cutting digits (Chelae).

Pedipalps : Also called palps or palpi, are paired, 4-segmented appendages, lateral to the hypostome and chelicerae. The segments are called articles.

Scutum : It is the dorsal chitinous shield found in hard ticks. In adult male ticks, it covers the entire dorsal surface except the capitulum while in adult females and nymphs, it is confined to a small area behind the capitulum.

Porose areas : They are paired depressed areas on the dorsal surface of basis capituli of adult female ticks and are believed to be sensory in function.

Punctations : These are circular dots or pits on the scutum which frequently bear hairs. The punctations may be coarse or fine, deep or shallow.

Eyes : They may be present as two small protuberances on the antero-lateral margin of the scutum as simple eyes.

Cervical groove : The term is applied to two grooves, which run backward from the inner angles of the scapulae of the scutum on either side.

Mammillae : In some of the soft ticks, the integument of the dorsum may show minute hemispherical or nipple-like protuberances called mammillae.

Haller's organ : A sensory organ located dorsally in the tarsi of the first pair of legs in hard ticks.

Genital pores : The genital openings in both male and female ticks are located behind the capitulum on the venter. Most of the females have two genital apertures. The prominent one is usually a transverse slit, which is located anteriorly on the ventral surface; serves for the exit of eggs and is called tocostome.

Anus : It is the terminal opening of the alimentary canal located postero-ventrally. In males it may be surrounded by chitinous plates.

Order : Parasitiformes
Suborder : Ixodida
Superfamily : Ixodoidea
Family : Argasidae

There is no dorsal shield or scutum. Mouthparts are ventral, not visible from the dorsal aspect in the nymphs and adults. Sexual dimorphism is not marked. They are commonly known as soft ticks.

Genus : *Argas*

Argas (Persicargas) persicus
(Plate : XXV)

Common name : Fowl tick. **Hosts** : Fowl, other domestic and wild birds including pigeons, ducks. **Habitat** : Adults and nymphs mostly hide in cracks and crevices of the poultry house during the day and visit their hosts for a short period during the night. **Distribution** : Cosmopolitan; freely distributed throughout India; more common in tropical and subtropical climates.

Size : Males measure 4 - 5 x 2.5 mm and females 7 - 10 x 5 – 6 mm. **Body** : Oval in outline; slightly narrower anteriorly and broader posteriorly; dorsoventrally flattened; slaty blue when engorged but yellowish brown when starved. Margin of the body is sharp and sutural line is well demarcated. The integument is wrinkled with numerous tiny folds and discs. **Capitulum** : Basis capitulum is rectangular with mouthparts hidden in the camerostome on the ventral surface. **Eyes** : Absent. **Spiracles** : In the form of oval plates, which are located between 3rd and 4th coxae. **Eggs** : Small, spherical, glistening yellow brown in colour and are laid in batches. **Larvae** :

Roughly circular body with six relatively long legs. Mouthparts are sub-terminal and unlike adults, are visible from dorsal aspect. Larvae may be found attached to the host, frequently under the wings. **Nymphs** : Have 4 pairs of legs, are smaller than adults and without sexual differentiation.

Economic importance : They worry their hosts at night and cause restlessness, anaemia, weight loss and even death. Some species may cause tick paralysis. They may also transmit avian spirochaetosis (*Borrelia anserina*) and aegyptianellosis (*Aegyptianella pullorum*) in birds.

Genus : *Ornithodoros*

O. savignyi

(Plate : XXV)

Common name : Eyed tampon or sand tampon. **Hosts** : Has preference for camels though it feeds on cattle, mules, pigs and even men. **Habitat** : Attacks the host for short periods to feed. **Distribution** : Arid parts of Africa, the Near East and India, common in southern Haryana.

Size : One of the largest species of ticks, measuring 5.0 - 12.0 x 4.0 - 8.5 cm. **Body** : Broad and rounded in front and is without sutural line. The integument is having innumerable minute elevations, known as mammillae. **Hypostome** : With well-developed teeth. **Eyes** : 2 pairs. **Eggs** : Laid in batches in the sand. **Larva** : Non-feeding until moulting to nymphal stage. **Nymph** : Several instars.

Economic importance : Many species cause tick worry, paralysis, anaemia and toxicosis leading to death particularly in calves, lambs and kids. *O. savignyi* may cause severe allergic reactions in man. *O. moubata* transmits relapsing fever (*Borrelia duttoni*) of man, African swine fever, Q fever

(*Coxiella burnetii*) in domestic animals and man; may also transmit avian spirochaetosis (*Borrelia anserina*) and aegyptianellosis (*Aegyptianella pullorum*) in fowls. *O. cariaceus* may transmit epizootic bovine abortion. *O. lahorensis* may transmit organisms of brucellosis and tularaemia in sheep. Similarly, *O. lahorensis* and *O. crossi* may also transmit *Trypanosoma evansi* mechanically.

Genus : *Otobius*

Otobius megnini

(Plate : XXV)

Common name : Spinose ear tick. **Hosts** : The larval and nymphal stages are parasitic in ears of dog, sheep, horse and cattle. **Distribution** : North and South America, Southern Africa and India.

Adults : Body narrow in the middle with a constriction at the middle and without spines. **Hypostome** : Vestigial and devoid of teeth. **Eggs** : Laid in sheltered spots of animal dwellings. **Larva** : Hexapod, measures 0.5 mm in length when unfed. Engorged larva is 3-4 mm. **Nymph** : Spiny, eight legged, measures 7-9 mm in length when fully grown. The body is widest at the middle and hypostome is well developed.

Economic importance : Nymphs cause marked irritation leading to inflammation and restlessness. There may be perforation of the ear drum and damage to the auricular nerve, leading to deafness. Death may occur in extreme cases.

Family : Ixodidae

The ticks belonging to this family possess a chitinous shield or scutum, which extends over the whole dorsal surface of the male and covers a small portion behind the head in larva, nymph and female. The mouthparts are anterior and well visible from the dorsal aspect. The adults have one pair of spiracles situated postero-laterally to the 4th coxae. They are commonly known as hard ticks.

Genus : *Ixodes*

(Plate : XXVI)

Many species are known of which some are found in India e.g. *Ixodes ovatus, I. acutitarsus, I. holocyclus* etc. **Hosts** : Most of the domestic animals, wild animals and man. **Distribution** : Cosmopolitan. Mainly confined to hilly areas in India.

Size : Comparatively small, males are 2.5 mm and females 3.5 mm, when unergorged. **Anal groove** : Distinct and surrounds the anus anteriorly (prostriate). **Eyes and festoons** : Absent. **Mouthparts** : Long, especially in females. Often the 2nd segment of the palp is constricted at the base, creating a gap between the palp and the hypostome. **Spiracular plates** : Oval in males and circular in females. **Ventral surface of male** : Has seven non-projecting, armor like plates.

Economic importance : Some species act as vectors of *Babesia divergens* of cattle, *Babesia microti* and Lyme disease (*Borrelia burgdorferi*) of man, *Anaplasma marginale*, *Ehrlichia phagocytophila*, *Coxiella burnetti*, tick-borne encephalitis and louping ill.

Genus : *Boophilus*

(Plate : XXVI)

Common name : Tropical cattle tick. **Hosts** : Primarily cattle but is also found on buffalo, horse, sheep, goat, camel, dog and deer. It is one-host tick. **Distribution** : Widely prevalent in Australia, West Indies, Mexico, Central and South America, South Africa, parts of Asia including India.

Size : Males are 2.0 x 1.0 mm and females 2.5 x 1.5 mm, when unengorged. **Anal groove** : Absent. **Eyes** : Present. **Festoons** : Absent. **Legs** : Coxa-I is triangular and bifid. **Mouthparts :** Hypostome and palpi are short. **Basis capitulum** : Hexagonal dorsally. **Plates of male** : Two adanal and two accessory shields, and a caudal appendage. **Eggs** : Average 4400 laid in a single batch in sheltered spots. **Larva** : Hexapod, feeds and moults on host's body. **Nymph** : Eight-legged. When engorged, appears slaty-gray in colour, feeds and moults on the host's body.

Economic importance : Acts as vector of babesiosis (*Babesia bigemina, B. argentina, B. bovis*), anaplasmosis (*Anaplasma marginale, A. centrale*) and rickettsial organisms (*Coxiella burnetti, Borrelia theileri*).

Genus : *Rhipicephalus*

(Plate : XXVI)

Rhipicephalus sanguineus

Common name : Brown dog tick. **Hosts** : Mainly on dogs, but occurs on a wide variety of mammals. It is a 3-host tick. **Distribution** : Cosmopolitan.

Size : Males are 2.25 mm and females 3.0 mm, when unengorged. **Anal groove** : Posterior. **Eyes and festoons** : Present. **Mouthparts** : Wider than long, hypostome and palpi are short. **Basis capitulum** : Hexagonal dorsally. **Coxa-I** : Deeply cleft and divided into large spurs. **Spiracles** : Comma-shaped, short in females, long in males. **Plates of male** : Adanal shields subtriangular.

Economic importance : Acts as vector of *Babesia canis*, *Hepatozoon canis* of dogs; *Babesia equi* and *B. caballi* of equines; *Ehrlichia canis* and *Rickettsia* spp.

Rhipicephalus haemaphysaloides

Hosts : Buffalo, cattle, camel, sheep, goat, horse, dog and wild animals. **Distribution** : Cosmopolitan.

Differs from *R. sanguineus* in the sickle-shaped anal plates of male, capitulum being as long as wide and is having 2 types of punctations i.e. large ones few and regularly arranged; smaller ones numerous and distributed all over the body.

Genus : *Haemaphysalis*

(Plate : XXVI)

There are numerous species, many of which are recorded in India.

Haemaphysalis bispinosa

Hosts : Cattle , buffalo and other ruminants, also equines. It is a 3-host tick. **Distribution** : Widely prevalent in various countries including India.

Size : Small. **Mouthparts** : Short and conical; article-II of palps has conspicuous lateral projection, which is more marked in females. **Basis capitulum**: Rectangular dorsally. **Coxae** : Each with a triangular pointed spur. **Festoons** : present. **Eyes** : Absent. **Anal plates of male** : Absent.

Economic importance : Acts as a vector of *Babesia gibsoni* and *Coxiella burnetti*.

Genus : *Hyalomma*

(Plate : XXVII)

Size : Large or medium. **Mouthparts** : Long (longirostrate). **Basis capitulum** : Subtriangular dorsally and long in relation to width. **Eyes** : Present. **Festoons** : Present but coalesced in certain cases. **Coxa-I** : Bifid in both sexes. **Anal plates of**

male : A pair of adanal shields, and in most cases a pair of accessory shields present. **Spiracles** : Comma-shaped in males and triangular in females.

Various species are described and the genus itself is often split into 3 subgenera viz. *Hyalommina*, *Hyalommasta* and *Hyalomma*. Ticks of the subgenus *Hyalommasta* parasitize tortoises and have no veterinary importance. Subgenus *Hyalomma* is characterized by coxa-I being deeply divided into narrow external spur and wider internal spur and additionally in the male, by the presence of a pair of well-developed chitinous protrusions (subanal shields). In species of subgenus *Hyalommina* the basis capitulum has lateral projections ventrally, adanal shields are very broad and subanal shields are absent.

Hyalomma anatolicum anatolicum

(Plate : XXVII)

Hosts : Usually two-host tick. Larvae and nymphs usually feed on small wild mammals and birds, while adults feed on domestic ruminants, horses and camels. **Distribution** : Parts of Middle East, Southern Russia to India.

Size : Males are small and narrow while females are of medium size. **Scutum**: Lightly punctated, with short but distinct lateral grooves. **Subanal shields** : Small, directly posterior to the adanal shields. **Genital operculum** : Usually circular in outline. **Eggs** : Average 3500, laid in a single batch. **Larva** : Hexapod, light yellowish brown in colour. **Nymph** : Eight legged, creamy white (unfed) to dark brown or gray (engorged).

Economic importance : Acts as vector of bovine tropical theileriosis (*Theileria annulata*), equine babesiosis (*B. equi*), Q fever (*Coxiella burnetti* and Crimean-Congo haemorrhagic fever.

H. dromedarii

Common name : Camel *Hyalomma.* **Hosts** : Cattle, camel and buffalo. **Distribution** : North Africa, Middle East to India.

Size : Larger than *H. a. anatolicum.* **Scutum** :Lateral grooves extend up to posterior third of the scutum. **Subanal shields** : Prominent, displaced laterally and not directly behind the adanal shields. **Genital operculum** : Elongated, triangular in outline. **Eggs** : Average 4500, laid in a single batch. **Larva** : Usually attaches on small mammals. **Nymph** : Frequently found engorging on camels. Slaty-gray in colour ; usually larger than the nymphs of *H. a. anatolicum.*

Economic importance : Acts as vector of bovine tropical theileriosis and harbours a number of viruses like Dera Ghazi Khan virus, Russian Summer Spring Encephalitis virus and Japanese Encephalitis virus etc.

Genus : *Amblyomma*

(Plate : XXVII)

Hosts : Three-host tick. The larvae and nymphs feed on rodents, rabbits and ground-inhabiting birds whereas the adults feed on cattle, deer, horse, sheep, carnivorous and reptiles.. **Distribution** : Tropical and sub-tropical areas of Africa, U.S.A., Mexico and South America. Has been recorded from India also.

Size : They are large sized ticks. The unfed females may be up to 8 mm in length and may reach 20 mm, when engorged. **Mouthparts** : Long i.e. much longer than the basis capitulum (longirostrate). The 2nd palpal segment is longer than the other segments. **Basis capitulum** : Subrectangular. **Eyes** : Present. **Scutum** : Ornate, has a bright pattern of coloured pigments. **Festoons** : Present. **Legs** : Have white pigment in rings at the far end of each segment. **Coxa-I** : Spurred. **Ventral plates in**

males : Absent, but small chitinous plaques may be present close to the festoons. **Eggs** : Up to 20,000, laid in a single batch.

Economic importance : Various species act as vector of heart-water disease (*Cowdria ruminantium*), Rocky Mountain spotted fever (*Rickettsia rickettsii*), tick-bite fever (*Rickettsia conori*), tularaemia (*Francisella tularensis*), Nairobi sheep disease (Nairovirus), Q fever (*Coxiella burnetti*), Lyme disease (*Borrelia burgdorferi*) etc.

Genus : *Dermacentor*

(Plate : XXVII)

Hosts : Most of the species are three-host ticks, while some are one-host ticks. The larvae and nymphs feed on small mammals especially rodents, whereas the adults feed on a number of domestic and wild animals, canines and also human-beings. **Distribution** : Asia including India, Europe, Mexico, Canada and America.

Size : Medium to large sized ticks. Males are 3 – 6 mm in length. The unfed females are 4 – 5 mm, while engorged females are 10 – 15 mm in length. **Mouthparts** : Short i.e. as long as basis capituli. **Basis capitulum** : Rectangular dorsally. **Eyes** : Present. **Scutum** : Ornate, has complex patterns of white pigment. **Festoons** : Present. **Coxa-I** : Bifid in both the sexes. Coxae – I to IV of males increase progressively in size; coxa – IV is the largest. . **Ventral plates/shields in males** : Absent. **Spiracular plates** : Sub-oval or comma shaped.

Economic importance : Various species act as vector of Rocky Mountain spotted fever (*Rickettsia rickettsii*), babesiosis (*Babesia bovis*, *B. caballi*, *B. canis*), bovine anaplasmosis (*Anaplasma marginale*), tularaemia (*Francisella tularensis*), Q fever (*Coxiella burnetti*), Colorado tick fever etc. They also cause tick-paralysis in their hosts.

Genus : *Nosomma*

Nosomma monstrosum

(Plate : XXVII)

Hosts : Mostly buffalo and preferred location is switch of the tail. **Distribution** : India, Nepal and extending to Indo-China.

Size : Medium. **Colour** : Dark brown. **Capitulum** : Has white and brown ornamentation superimposed. **Basis capitulum** : Rectangular, about twice as broad as long in males but with equal length-breadth in females. **Palps** : Short and broad. Article II is heavily ornate in males. In females, article III is subtriangular. **Hypostome** : With dental formula 3/3. **Scutum and legs** : Ornate. **Eyes** : Flat. **Festoons** : Present. **Spiracles** : Comma shaped with short, broad tail in male and subtriangular in female. **Male venter** : Has adanal and trilobed subanal shields but no accessory shields. **Genital aperture** : On level with coxa-II in both male and female.

Economic importance : Not known.

MITES

They are much smaller in size than ticks. Hypostome when present, is without teeth. A number of species are parasitic on domestic animals and poultry.

ORDER : PARASITIFORMES

Suborder : Gamasida (=Mesostigmata)

Body is like that of ticks, divided into two portions, the anterior small is called gnathosoma, which bears the mouthparts, and the posterior is idiosoma. Single pair of stigmata are lateral and outside the coxae of the legs. The mites are comparatively large, ranging from 0.2 - 2.5 mm in length.

Family : Dermanyssidae

Genus : *Dermanyssus*

Dermanyssus gallinae

(Plate : XXVIII)

Common name : Red mite of poultry. **Hosts** : Fowl, pigeon, sparrow and other caged birds. **Location** : Nymphs and adults are periodic blood suckers and like *Argas* can be located in cracks and crevices. **Distribution** : Cosmopolitan.

Size : The engorged female is about 1 mm long (or larger), visible to unaided eye especially when freshly fed on blood, the male being smaller, about 0.75 mm. **Chelicerae** : Long and needle like. **Dorsal shield** : Truncated posteriorly and does not reach the posterior extremity in female : **Anal plate** : Large and bears 3 setae. **Genito-ventral plate** : Rounded posteriorly and bears one pair of setae. **Spiracles**: In the middle of the body, behind coxa-III. **Eggs** : Laid usually after a blood meal, in dark, sheltered spots, in batches of up to seven pearly white, elliptical eggs. **Larva** : Hexapod, non-feeding. **Nymphs** : Two stages i.e. proto and deuto, feeding on the host's blood. Each feeding lasts 24-48 hours.

Economic importance : When in large numbers, they may cause reduced egg production, loss of body weight and even death due to exsanguination.

Family : Macronyssidae

Genus : *Ornithonyssus*

Ornithonyssus* (=*Liponyssus*) *bursa

(Plate : XXVIII)

Common name : Tropical fowl mite. **Hosts** : Fowl, pigeon, sparrow and other birds. **Location** : Found mostly on fluff of feathers especially on those around the vent. **Distribution** : Warmer or tropical countries including India.

Dorsal plate : Tapers gradually to a blunt posterior end. **Chelicerae of female** : Long and whip-like but not needle-like. **Anal plate** : Egg-shaped, bears the anus on the anterior half. **Spiracles** : As in *Dermanyssus*. **Eggs** : May be found in the fluff of the feathers as well as in the nests of the birds. **Larvae** : Hexapod, non-feeding, moult in less than 24 hours. **Nymphs** : Two stages i.e. proto and deuto, occur on the host body.

Economic importance : Same as of *D. gallinae*.

Suborder : Acaridida (=Astigmata)

They are small, thin-skinned mites lacking obvious shields. The coxae are sunk into the body and are known as epimeres. True-paired claws are absent.

Family : Sarcoptidae

Genus : *Sarcoptes*

Sarcoptes scabiei

(Plate : XXVIII)

Common name : Scabies mite or itch mite. **Hosts** : Man and a number of different domestic and wild mammals. **Distribution** : Cosmopolitan. **Habitat** : Found more or less deeply burrowed in skin.

Size : Minute mites; female measures 0.33-0.45 mm x 0.35 mm, the males are smaller, 0.2-0.24 mm x 0.15-0.2 mm. **Shape** : Roughly circular in outline. **Colour** : Dirty white, translucent. **Dorsal surface** : Covered with fine folds and grooves and bears a number of small triangular scales. **Mouthparts** : Have a pair of minute chelicerae and 3-jointed pedipalps. **Legs** : All the 4-

pair of legs are short and the 3rd and 4th pairs do not project beyond the body margin. The tarsi of the 1st, 2nd and 4th pair of legs in the male and the 1st and 2nd pair of legs in the female end in bell-shaped suckers, other legs ending in bristles. The pedicels bearing these suckers are not segmented. **Eggs** : Oval, 40-50 in number, are laid in the tunnel burrowed by the female. **Larva** : Six-legged, tiny creature. **Nymphs** : Two stages, proto and deuto nymphs. They have four pair of legs but no genital aperture.

Economic importance : Zoonotic in nature; severe infestation leads to loss of condition in animals and even death, when spread all over the body.

Family : Knemidocoptidae (= Cnemidoptidae)

Genus : *Knemidocoptes* (= *Cnemidopcoptes*)

Knemidocoptes mutans

(Plate : XXVIII)

Common name : Scaly leg mite of poultry. **Hosts** : Mostly fowl and turkeys but other birds are also susceptible. **Location** : In the skin underneath the scales of legs. **Distribution** : Cosmopolitan, common in India.

In general, these mites resemble *Sarcoptes scabiei* but striae on the dorsal surface are interrupted by scales, appearing as raised sculptures. There are no spines on the dorsal surface. All legs of males bear stalked caruncles (suckers) while the legs of females and nymphs are devoid of suckers.

Economic importance : Large populations result in deformation of the scale structure on the legs of birds with frequent crippling and deformity.

K. gallinae

Common name : Depluming itch mite. **Hosts** : Poultry, pheasants and geese. **Location** : In the skin along the shaft of feathers. **Distribution** : Cosmopolitan, but not common in India.

This mite differs from *K. mutans* in not having raised sculptures on the dorsal surface.

Family : Psoroptidae

Genus : *Psoroptes*

Psoroptes ovis

(Plate : XXIX)

Common name : Sheep scab mite. **Hosts** : Sheep and cattle. **Distribution** : Cosmopolitan.

Size : Males measure 0.45 - 0.60 mm x 0.30 - 0.37 mm and ovigerous females, 0.53 - 0.75 x 0.30 - 0.37 mm. **Body** : Oval, the dorsal surface is devoid of scales and spines. **Legs** : All the four pairs of legs are long and visible from dorsal aspect. Males have tarsal suckers with long, 3-jointed pedicels on 1st, 2nd and 3rd pair of legs while in females, the 1st, 2nd and 4th pair of legs bear such suckers and the 3rd pair has long setae instead of suckers. **Accessory features** : Males have a pair of prominent adanal suckers on the ventral aspect and a pair of copulatory tubercles. Pubescent female is provided with a pair of copulatory tubercles posteriorly, which get lost as it becomes ovigerous. **Eggs** : Measure 0.25 mm in length and are laid on the skin of the host at the edge of active lesions. They are oval, glistening white in colour. **Larva** : Measures 0.33 mm, long with all legs terminating in setae. **Nymphs** : There are two nymphal stages, proto and deuto. Nymphs maturing earlier usually develop into females.

Economic importance : In heavy infestation, there is loss of fleece and markedly reduced wool production.

Genus : *Chorioptes*

Chorioptes bovis

(Plate : XXIX)

Common name : Chorioptic mange mite. **Hosts** : Cattle, horse, sheep and goat. **Distribution** : Cosmopolitan.

This mite resembles *Psoroptes ovis* except that the tarsal suckers have unjointed pedicels. Suckers are present on all the legs in males and on the 1st, 2nd and 4th pair of legs in the females. They are comparatively smaller in size.

Economic importance : In horses, they cause severe itching and irritation on the lower parts of the legs and reduce their performance. In cattle, they cause lesions at the base of the tail, on the perineum, feet, hind legs, udder and scrotum.

Genus : *Otodectes*

Otodectes cynotis

(Plate : XXIX)

Common name : Ear mange mite of dogs. **Hosts** : Domestic and wild canids. **Location** : Deep in the auditory canal of ear. **Distribution** : Cosmopolitan.

Morphologically this mite resembles *Chorioptes* except that 4th pair of legs in females is small. In males, neither the copulatory suckers are prominent nor are the abdominal lobes marked.

Economic importance : These mites generally live deep in the ear canal and may cause convulsions in heavily infested dogs and cats.

Suborder : Prostigmata

They vary in size from 100 μm to 16 mm, are weakly sclerotized and where there is an internal respiratory system, the stigmata open on the gnathosoma or anterior part of the propodosoma. The chelicerae may be blade-like or styletiform, rarely chelate. The coxae of the legs may be incorporated into the ventral surface of the body or may be united.

Family : Demodicidae

Genus : *Demodex*

(Plate : XXIX)

Common name : Follicle mite. **Hosts** : Man, dog, sheep, goat, cattle and pig. **Distribution** : Cosmopolitan.

Size : Female measures 0.35 - 0.4 mm, male slightly smaller. **Body** : Elongate, worm-like, divisible into head, thorax and a prolonged abdomen bearing rings or striations. **Mouthparts** : Consist of a pair of chelicerae, a hypostome and a pair of spiracular openings on the ventral side of the capitulum near its base.

Legs : Very short, 4 pairs in adults and nymphs and 3 pairs in larvae. **Eggs** : Spindle shaped, 20-24 in numbers, laid in the hair follicles. **Larva and nymph** : Found at the mouth of the follicle to which they are swept by the sebaceous flow.

Economic importance : It causes formation of nodules and pustules in its hosts. Due to secondary infections particularly in dogs, mortality may occur.

Family : Trombiculidae

They are the largest known mites. Due to dense pilose setae on legs, body and to some extent on palps of nymphs and adults, they are called velvet mites.

Genus : *Leptotrombidium*

(Plate : XXIX)

Common name : Scrub itch mite. **Distribution** : *L. akamushi* is distributed in Japan and China while *L. deliense* also includes Indian sub-continent in its range.

Hosts : Insectivorous, rodents; also man, cattle and carnivorous. **Adults** : Found in soil or as predators on soft-bodied insects. The nymphs and adults are also known as velvet mites. **Eggs** : Spherical. **Larva** : Hexapod, about 250-400 mm in size. It has blade-like chelicerae; situated anterio-medially, which are flanked by segmented palps. The penultimate segment of palps bears a claw and thc terminal segment bears ciliated setae. A scutum is present dorsally, which bears 5 ciliated setae.

Economic importance : The larva is parasitic on vertebrates and may also act as vector of scrub typhus in man (*Rickettsia tsutsugamushi*).

Techniques involved in the study of arthropods

While studying arthropods/arthropod infestations there are some techniques, which need description. A few of such techniques, as given below, have been described in detail.

1. Collection of arthropods
2. Transportation of arthropods
3. Storage of arthropods
4. Dry mounting of arthropods
5. Preparation of permanent slides of arthropods
6. Collection and identification of skin scrapings for the mites.

Collection of arthropods

Arthropods are collected from the field with the following objectives :

i) To have their proper identification and location etc.

ii) To know their prevalence and population density in a particular area.

iii) To demonstrate their identifying features to the students, farmers and field veterinarians.

iv) To rear them in the laboratory for carrying out research/ to evolve their strategic control programmes/to know their potential significance to animal as well as human health.

Arthropods vary in their habitat while affecting animals and human beings. Some are found flying in the vicinity of animals and human beings and in their dwelling places, some are seen permanently attached to the body of their hosts while some are found inhabiting on the walls, in the cracks and crevices of houses, in the beddings, in the skirting, in the wooden framework of wall posters, on the ground and even on the grass blades in the pasture land etc.

For collection of these arthropods from their variable habitats the different kinds of devices are employed, which include:

i) Insect net

ii) Aspirator

iii) Trap

iv) Tick drag

v) Berlese funnel

vi) Manual means

i) Insect net : This device is used for collecting the flying arthropods. Flying insects are swept from the dwellings of animals/humans as well as from their vicinity and are contained in a suitable container (Plate : XXX).

ii) Aspirator : It is a special kind of device used for collecting arthropods sitting on the walls or inhabiting in the cracks and crevices, skirting, wooden frameworks of wall posters etc. (Plate : XXX). This device consists of a suitable container fitted with two tubes (glass or rubber). One tube is placed on the arthropod sitting on the wall or near the opening of the crack or crevice while through other tube the vacuum is created in the container so that the arthropods are sucked up in the container.

iii) Trap : Various kinds of traps may also be employed in the field say in the animal sheds/dwellings for collecting flies, fleas, ticks etc. (Plate : XXX). A few such traps are as follows:

a) Malaise trap : Widely used for trapping the dipteran flies.

b) Manning trap : Used for sampling of Tabanids.

c) The New Jersey light trap : Quite useful for capturing mosquitoes.

d) Carbon dioxide burrow trap : It contains dry ice and is used for collecting ticks and fleas from animal burrows (Plate : XXXI).

These traps contain some attractants so that the insects may be attracted and trapped. The attractants may be host, light, baits etc. These traps be can fixed at suitable places and the arthropods can easily be collected.

iv) Tick drag : This device is used for collecting the tick larvae/nymphs or even adult ticks crawling on the grass blades in the pasture land. It is made up of one sq. meter flannel (lint) like cloth material fitted on its one side with 1.2 meter long draw bar (Plate : XXXI).

This device is dragged over the grass in the grazing pastures and the crawling stages of ticks stick to the underside of the cloth from where they are collected.

v) Berlese funnel : It is used to separate fleas from beddings or bugs from nests or mites from debris. This apparatus consists of a funnel in whose broader end a sieve is fitted. The material like grass/litter/wool from which insects are to be separated is kept on the sieve. A light source is usually provided above the sieve. The insects will move downwards through the sieve and can be collected in a collecting jar, kept at the bottom of the assembly (Plate : XXXI).

vi) Manual means : Certain arthropods can be collected directly from the body of the host or from the ground. These include lice, mites, fleas, ticks, maggots etc. Such arthropods are collected manually with the help of forceps or even by hands.

Lice and fleas can be searched on the body of the hosts by parting the hairs, wool or feathers and on spotting they are directly picked up with the help of forceps into the containers.

Adult ticks and their developmental stages while feeding on the animals remain attached by keeping their mouthparts embedded into the skin. They should be removed gently and care should be taken that no mouthpart may break, as these help in identification.

Mites remain embedded either superficially or deep into the skin of their hosts and can be collected by taking the skin scrapings.

Transportation of arthropods

After collection, the arthropods are to be carried to the laboratory. Most of the arthropods are rapidly susceptible to heat and desiccation. To avoid this, the arthropods are usually transported as living specimens through some means in a relatively cool and moist environment.

Arthropods should be carried in proper containers like plastic/stopper vials. Such containers must have the provision of aeration. In case of stopper vials, the stopper should be of simple cork or it should have one hole covered by a fine mesh cloth (muslin cloth). There are many means for transporting arthropods but the best ones are as under :

For shorter distances, the arthropods can be transported simply in plastic vials containing paper labelling and moistened filter paper. Such vials can easily be carried in shirt pockets as the perspiration of body provides the needed cooling protection. For longer distances, the safer technique is that the vials should be prepared before the collecting trip. In this case the stopper vials should be used. For preparation of vials, a mixture is prepared by mixing one part of charcoal powder with nine parts of gypsum (plaster of Paris). By adding water to this mixture, a thick slurry is made. A layer of this slurry is to be made at the bottom of each such vial. After collecting the arthropods in these vials, the vials should be stoppered. Occasionally, a few drops of water are added to the hardened bottom layer in the vials and in doing so the water vapours are released slowly and the moist environment is maintained.

For certain dipterans, the cloth cages on wooden or wire frames are used and the whole cage is to be covered with some material kept moistened with water.

Storage of arthropods in the laboratory

For temporary storage, the arthropods can best be stored at cool temperatures. Store them in an ice-filled thermos bottle or in B.O.D. incubator e.g. ticks can easily be stored at 17-18 ^{o} C. If the arthropods are to be stored for longer duration then they are to be stored in suitable wet preservatives or as dry mountants.

Wet preservatives : The most commonly used wet preservatives are either 70% ethyl alcohol or 10% formalin. Ethyl alcohol is preferred over formalin. Alcohol usually evaporates during the period of preservation and to check the same, 2-3 drops of glycerin should be poured over the alcohol. Glycerin forms a layer at the top and prevents evaporation of the preservative. The arthropods (living specimens) being brought to laboratory are transferred to glass bottles (Reagent bottles) containing the suitable preservative and are then stored.

There are certain arthropods, which are identified by their natural colours like blowflies. If these flies are to be preserved in wet preservatives, discoloration occurs in longer duration. To maintain their natural colour such arthropods are preserved either as dry mountants or if at all wet preservatives are to be used then few drops of chloroform are added.

Dry mounting : In this technique the living arthropods collected from the field are to be killed in killing jars and then mounted as dry by pinning them with the help of entomological pins. Through this technique the optimal natural form and color of arthropods is preserved.

The detailed technique is as follows :

I. Killing of arthropods :

The living specimens before being pinned are to be killed. For killing the arthropods, special type of jars or other suitable containers can be prepared or can be purchased from the market. Such devices include :

A. Killing jars : Such jars are available with most of the biological supply houses or can be made at our own at very little expense. In killing jars a variety of materials releasing toxic gas may be used. Usually granular salt of potassium cyanide or sodium cyanide and even insecticidal fumigant like DDVP (dichlorvos) are used.

Such jars contain a bottom layer of toxic material covered with 1.2 cm layer of dry sawdust, which is again over-covered by 0.6 cm thick layer of plaster of Paris. Such jars can be used for several months without making any change in it. The arthropods are placed over the top layer of plaster of Paris and the jar is kept air tight (Plate XXXII).

B. Improved killing technique : Arthropods can also be made killed by some other improvised devices like :

a) A cotton swab soaked in anaesthetic like chloroform or ether is placed at the bottom of large test tube or jar. Some paper strips are placed over the swab. The specimens are dropped over these paper strips and the container is covered with a tight-fitting blotting paper disk.

b) Arthropods can also be killed by simply keeping them over dry ice contained in a suitable insulated container.

II. Mounting of arthropods :

The killed specimens are mounted as dry, for which the following techniques are used :

a) Pinning of arthropods : Here the freshly killed arthropods are pinned directly by using entomological pins. Large sized and soft-bodied arthropods can easily be pinned. The large entomological pin is inserted through the thorax slightly to the right of midline (Plate : XXXII). The small sized arthropods can be mounted on small entomological pins, which are known as "minuten nadeln". Usually the dipterans and hymenopterans are mounted by this technique (Plate : XXXII).

b) Mounting on card board : Usually the minute sized arthropods or the hardened and brittle ones are mounted in this way. Certain card points are cut and the freshly killed specimens are glued directly onto the tip of card points. The base of the card point is inserted with the pin (it may be entomological pin or an ordinary alpine).

In both kinds of mounts, the proper labelling (identification, place of collection, date, name of collector, host involved etc.) is very essential.

The pinned arthropods (may be on entomological pins or on card points) can best be displayed either in insect boxes or museum cases (Plate : XXXII). The base of such boxes or cases is having a layer of wax and pinned arthropods can well be fixed in this layer. The individual pinned arthropods can also be stored in test tubes of suitable sizes. Such tubes should be stoppered with cork and the pinned arthropods can well be inserted on the underside of the cork (Plate : XXXII). Such tubes can further be placed in wide mouthed bottles containing cotton at the base.

Preparation of permanent slides of arthropods

In this technique the arthropods are mounted on the glass slides in a suitable medium. This is again a method of preserving the arthropods for their identification.

Large sized arthropods are difficult to be mounted as whole. For such specimens if whole mount is needed then dry mount is the best technique. If they are to be mounted on the slides then their various body parts, provided with identifying morphological features, are to be dissected out with the help of dissecting needles/scalpel under the dissecting microscope. Such body parts may be wings, antennae, mouthparts, legs etc. Their developmental stages may be mounted as whole specimens or if they happen to be of large size then again the body regions with identifying salient features like anterior and posterior spiracles of larvae are separated and processed further.

The small sized arthropods like ticks, mites, fleas, lice etc. can be mounted as whole.

For mounting purpose, the hard bodied (heavily sclerotized or blood engorged) specimens like ticks may be made clear and soft first. For this, it is advisable to place them in aqueous 10% solution of potassium hydroxide for few hours at room temperature. The time period may be reduced if the said solution is warmed. For blood-engorged specimens it is suggested that they should be pricked with the help of dissecting needle at various places along their lateral margins and while in solution they should gently be pressed with the help of camel hair brush from time to time. After clearing, these specimens are to be removed of potassium hydroxide by gently washing them in tap water and then these are either transferred to 70% alcohol (C_2H_5OH) or may directly be processed for mounting.

These various separated body parts or the whole cleared specimens whatever the case may be, are mounted on glass slides in suitable mounting medium or mountant. Various kinds of mountants, as listed below can be used :

i) Glycerin

ii) Hoyer's medium

iii) Canada balsam

iv) DPX medium

i) Mounting in glycerin : Glycerin is usually used as a temporary mountant. In this medium the arthropods remain preserved only for a short duration say a few days. For mounting in glycerin the specimens can directly be mounted on glass slides without any dehydration. The specimens from water or 70% alcohol are put on the glass slide in the centre. The medium is poured over the slide dipping the specimen. Pouring of medium is carried slowly and entangling of air bubbles in between is avoided. Afterwards cover the dipped specimen with a suitable sized cover slip.

ii) Mounting in Hoyer's medium : This medium is considered to be the best medium for the preparation of permanent slides of the arthropods as the arthropod specimens can be preserved for long duration. The mountant is available in the market but can also be prepared in the laboratory according to the following constituents in definite proportions : gum Arabic = 60 parts, glycerin = 40 parts, chloral hydrate = 100 parts and thymol = 1 part. This medium is also known as "gum Arabic medium". While mounting the arthropods in this medium the specimens should be preserved in 70% alcohol first and then these are to be transferred in 50% glycerin and afterwards they can be directly mounted in the medium on the glass slides as given in case of glycerin medium above. Like glycerin mountant, this medium also does not require dehydration of arthropods except in 70% alcohol.

iii) Mounting in Canada balsam : Canada balsam is also a suitable mountant for permanent mount of the arthropods. This medium is available in the market. The disadvantage of this medium is that the mounting of arthropods in this medium is a cumbersome process as the specimens need dehydration and clearing before being mounted.

The specimens are to be dehydrated through ascending grades of ethyl alcohol i.e. 70%, 80%, 90%, 95% and absolute i.e. the arthropods are transferred to successive grades of alcohol and are left for 20-30 minutes in each grade. Afterwards they are to be cleared in a clearing agent. Different clearing agents may be used i.e. eugenol, xylol, cellusolve, beech wood creosote or cedar wood oil. Out of these, cedar wood oil is preferred. This agent is available in the market but sometimes it is very thick and viscous fluid so it may be made thin by mixing it with xylene. The specimens are immersed in this clearing agent for a few hours till they become transparent and clear. After clearing, the specimens are finally mounted in Canada balsam onto the glass slides as per procedure given in case of glycerin medium.

iv) Mounting in DPX medium : DPX mountant is also available in the market and is used for the preparation of permanent slides of the arthropods. This medium like Canada balsam also needs dehydration and clearing of the specimens before being mounted but it is being preferred over Canada balsam. The method of mounting the arthropods in this medium is the same as in case of Canada balsam.

Hardening of mountant

Whatever the mountant is used for the preparation of permanent slides, it is to be hardened. Hardening of mountant in the freshly prepared slides can be carried out by keeping the slides on a smooth and horizontal surface for drying at ordinary room temperature but it takes longer period, a month or so, which can be reduced to a week or more, if the slides are kept warm at 40 °C.

Labelling of permanent slides

After the mountant is hardened, the slides are to be labelled. The mountant on the periphery of cover slips or over the cover slips is to be removed and can best be achieved with the help of xylene. Then on one side of the slide a label is placed quoting the name of arthropod or body part. Such slides are stored properly in suitable container for which slide boxes of different sizes may be used.

Collection and identification of skin scrapings for parasitic mites

Skin scrapings are taken from the animals suspected to be suffering from mite infestations or 'mange'. Different mites, which infest the animals as well as birds are *Sarcoptes, Psoroptes, Demodex, Otodectes, Notoedres, Cnemidocoptes* spp. etc. These mites infest different body parts of their hosts i.e. some are found burrowing deep into the skin like *Sarcoptes*, *Demodex* and *Notoedres* while others infest superficially.

The technique involved for demonstrating the mites, is the examination of skin scrapings, as given below :

The mites infested lesion is sclected and the hairs over the edge of the lesion are clipped. Then take a Petri plate of suitable size and a scalpel. The scalpel blade and the rim of the Petri plate should be coated first with an oily substance, which may be liquid paraffin or vaseline. Then scrape the skin over the edge gently and take the material in the Petri plate. This process should be continued till a slight amount of blood oozes out. This is done in order to contain the deep-seated mites, if any. Cover the Petri plate with its lid and bring the material in the laboratory and examine it. The skin scrapings can be examined by the following ways :

I. Direct examination : Put the Petri plate containing the skin scrapings directly under the stereoscope and look for mites. The mites, if present can be spotted by their movements within the scrapings or the Petri plate can be heated a little and then the movements may be observed. Another way is to take a small amount of skin scrapings on a glass slide and pour 2-3 drops of liquid paraffin over it, cover it with cover slip and examine under suitable magnification of microscope.

II. Examination after boiling : If mites are not seen by direct examination, the scrapings are boiled in 5-10% of potassium hydroxide solution (caustic potash) for 5-10 minutes. The boiling in caustic potash is carried to clear the material of debris which usually dissolves in this solution. The material is then centrifuged a little and the sediment is then examined on a glass slide under the microscope.

III. Examination after mounting in permanent slide preparation : If mites are present in the material, these can also be mounted on slides permanently. For this purpose the material is cleared of debris by boiling in caustic potash solution as above. Then give washings to the sediment in water for 2-3 times to remove caustic potash. Afterwards the sediment is to be dehydrated in ascending grades of alcohol and then cleared in clearing agent in the same way as described for the preparation of permanent slides of arthropods. Since the mites are microscopic in size so the centrifugation is carried out at each stage. Finally from the clearing agent the sediment containing the mites is mounted in a suitable mountant in the same way as described for preparation of permanent slides of arthropods.

The mounting medium to be used for mites can be :

(a) Hoyer's medium

(b) Berlese fluid : This medium can be prepared in the laboratory. Dissolve 13 gm of gum Arabic in 20 ml of distilled water. Now add 10 ml of glucose syrup and 5 ml of acetic acid to it. The whole mixture is then saturated with chloral hydrate up to 100 gm. Allow the mixture to settle for one to two weeks and then the mixture is ready for use.

(c) Jelly medium : This can also be prepared in the laboratory according to the following constituents : Gelatin = 20 parts, Glycerin = 100 parts, Carbolic acid = 120 parts, Distilled water = 2 parts.

(d) DPX mountant : This medium is available in the market and is used as such.

After mounting in medium, the slides are dried, the medium on outside of cover slip is removed and the slides are ringed.

Ringing of slides : The slide with mounted mites is kept on a ringing table and the edges of the cover slip are ringed with the help of nail polish. A brush dipped in nail polish is kept over the rim of the cover slip and the slide is rotated on the ringing table. In this way the edges of the cover slip are ringed from all sides. Ringing prevents the medium from drying for a longer period. The cover slips used for mounting of mites are usually the round ones.

ILLUSTRATIONS

PLATE I

Fig. 1: Wing of *Tabanus* showing various wing-veins

a – costa, b – subcosta, c – squama, d – antisquama, e – alula, f – anal lobe, A – anal veins, Cu – cubital veins, M – medial veins, R – radial veins

Fig. 2: Wing of *Musca* showing various wing-veins and cells

a – costa, b – subcosta, c – squama, d – antisquama, e – alula, f – discal cell, g – cubital cell, h – medial cell, i – apical cell, j – radial cell, A – anal veins, Cu – cubital veins, M – medial veins, R – radial veins

Fig. 3: Wing of *Tabanus* showing various cross veins

a – humeral cross-vein, b – anterior cross-vein, c – radio-medial cross- vein, d – inter-radial cross-vein, e – posterior cross-vein, f – medio-cubital cross-vein

PLATE I

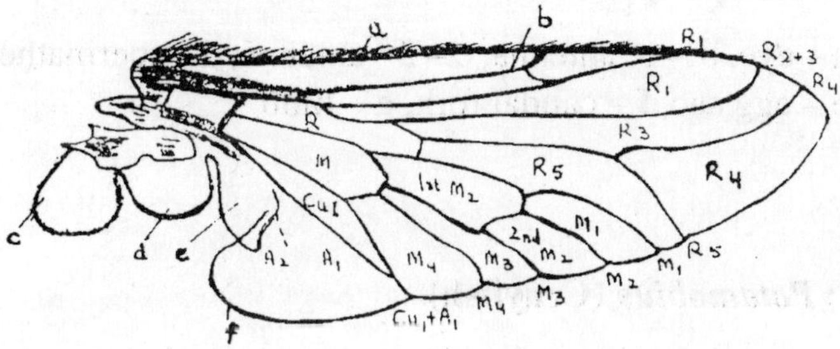

Fig. 1

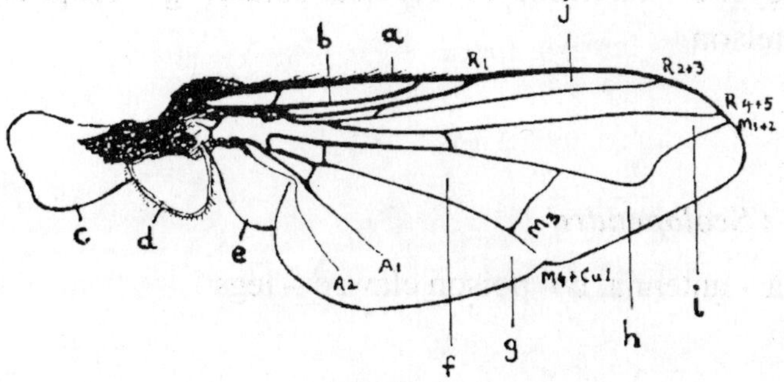

Fig. 2

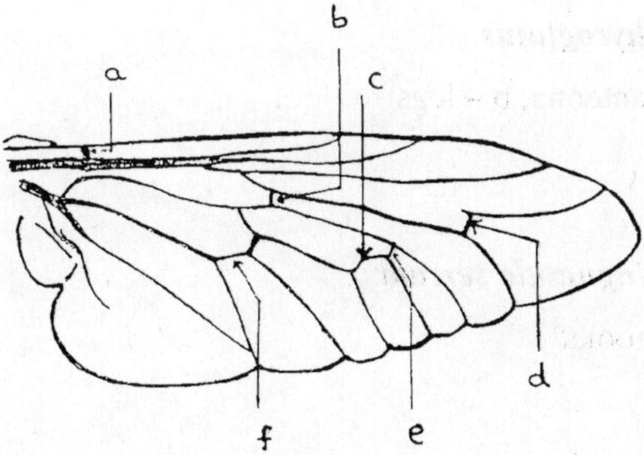

Fig. 3

PLATE II

Fig. 1 : *Cyclops* spp.

a – eye, b – 1st antenna, c – 2nd antenna, d – spermatheca, e – egg sac, f – caudal fork, g – limb

Fig. 2 : *Potamobius* (Crayfish)

a – antenna, b – cheliped, c – antennule, d – compound eye, e – rostrum, f – cervical suture, g – uropod, h – telson

Fig. 3 : *Scolopendra*

a – antenna, b – poison claw, c – legs

Fig. 4 : *Thyroglutus*

a – antenna, b – legs

Fig. 5 : *Linguatula serrata*

a - hooks

PLATE II

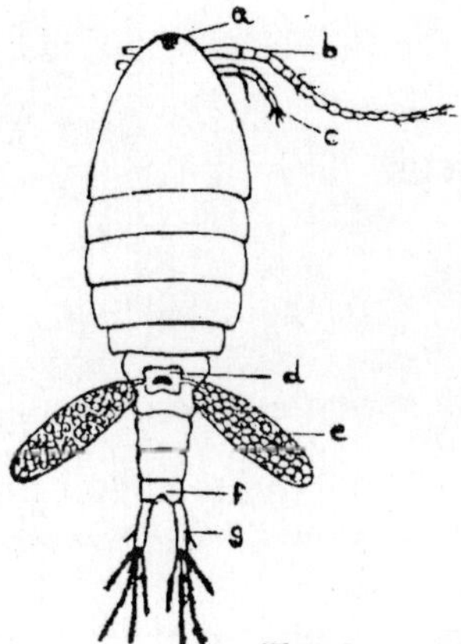

Fig. 1

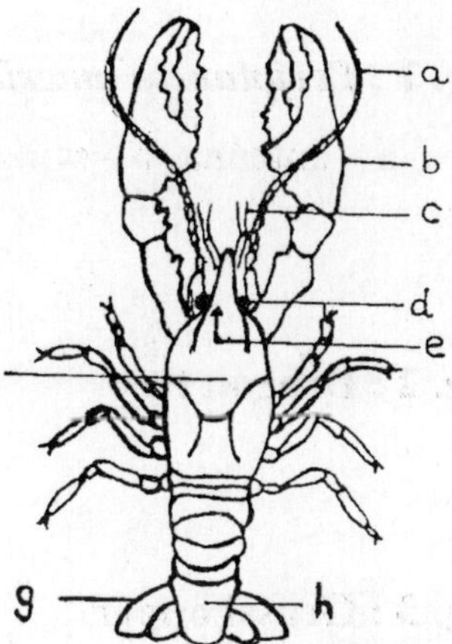

Fig. 2

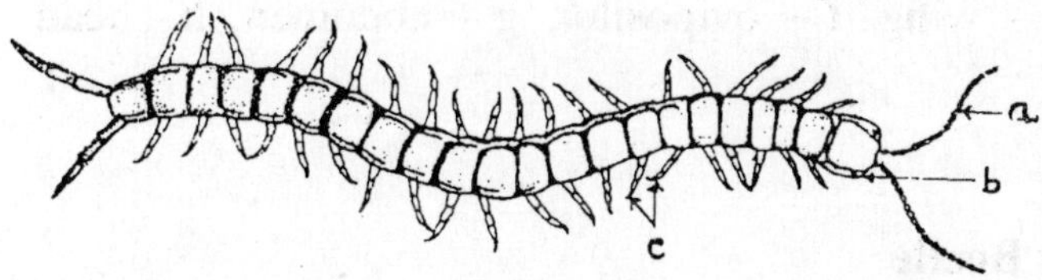

Fig. 3

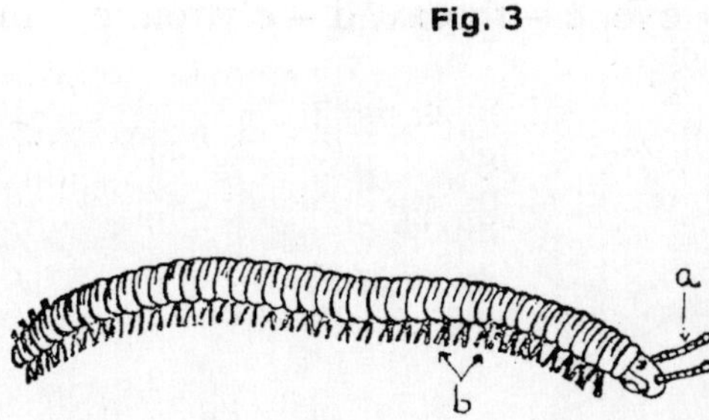

Fig. 4

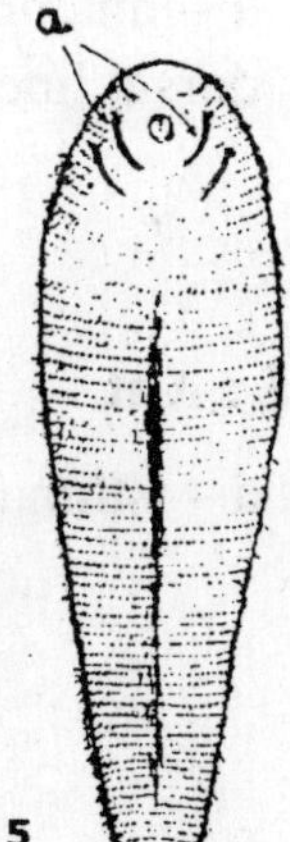

Fig. 5

PLATE III

Fig. 1 : *Periplaneta americana*

a – antenna, b – wing, c – cercus

Fig. 2 : Dragon fly

Fig. 3 : Grasshopper

a – antenna, b – compound eye, c – thorax, d – leg, e – wing, f – ovipositor, g – abdomen, h – head

Fig. 4 : Beetle

a – antenna, b – eye, c – thorax, d – elytron, e – mid dorsal line

Fig. 5 : Ant

a – isthmus

PLATE III

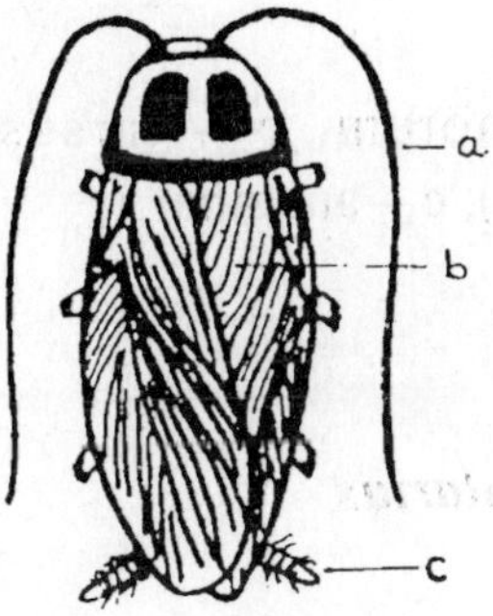

Fig. 1

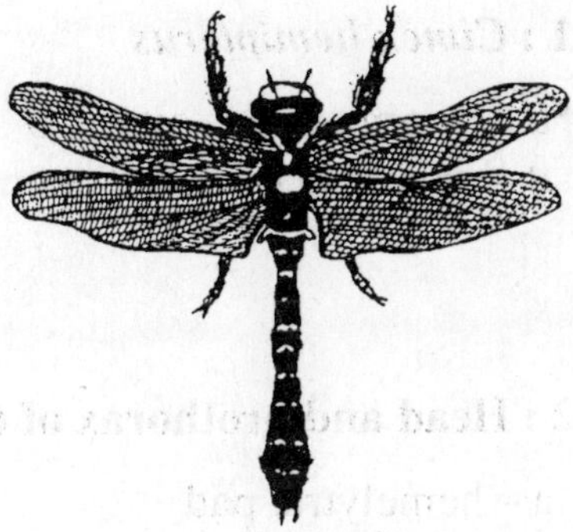

Fig. 2

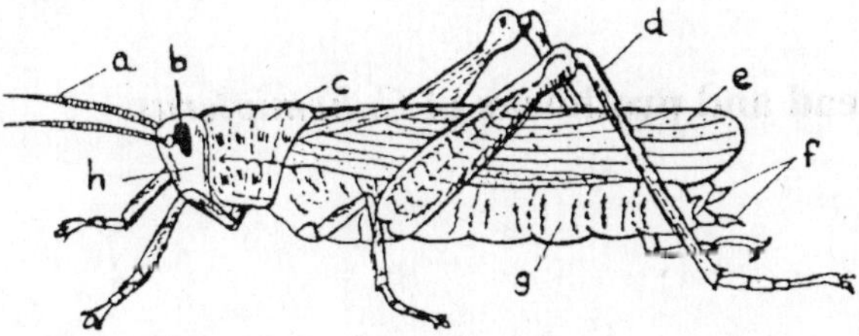

Fig. 3

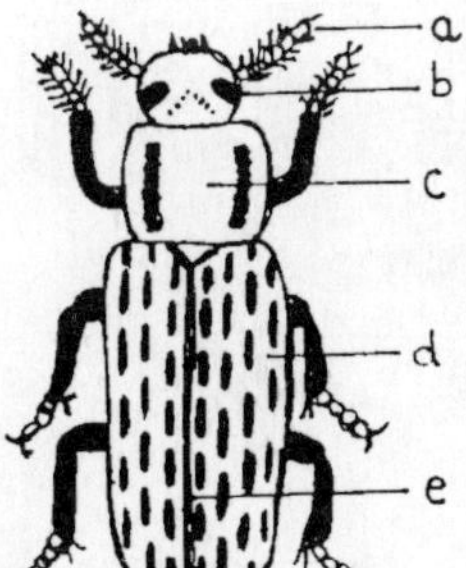

Fig. 4

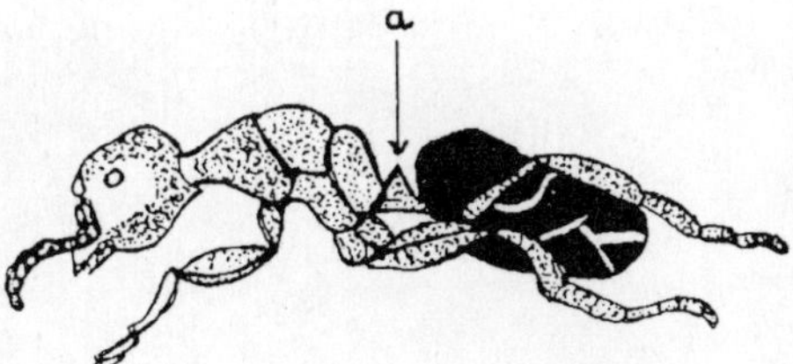

Fig. 5

PLATE IV

Fig. 1 : *Cimex hemipterus*

a – compound eye, b – pronotum, c – tarsus, d – copulatory orifice (spermalage), e – antenna

Fig. 2 : Head and prothorax of *C. lectularius*

a – hemelytral pad

Fig. 3 : Head and prothorax of *C. hemipterus*

PLATE IV

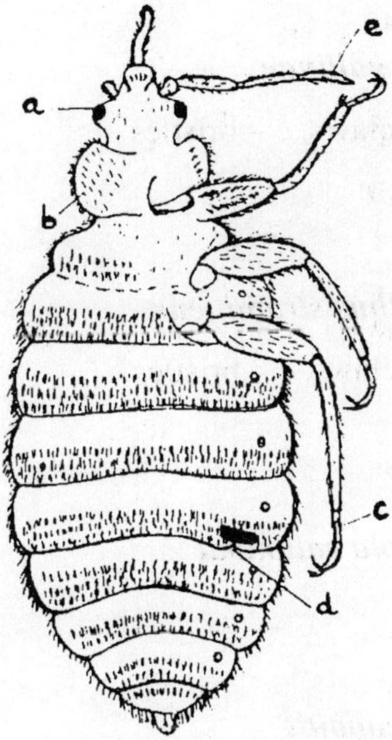

Fig. 1

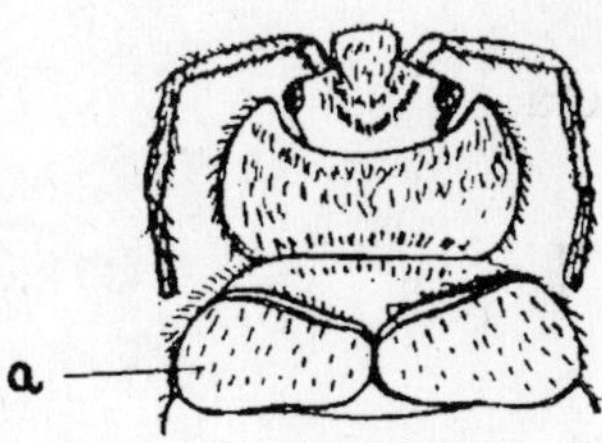

Fig. 2

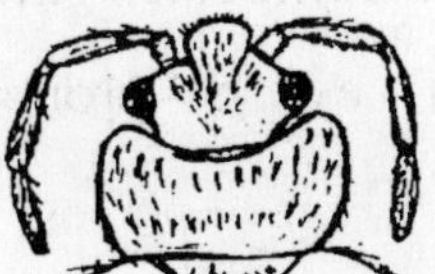

Fig. 3

PLATE V

Fig. 1 : ***Menopon gallinae***

a – eye, b – claws, c – bristles

Fig. 2 : ***Menacanthus stramineus***

a – eye, b – claws, c – bristles

Fig. 3 : ***Columbicola columbae***

Fig. 4 : ***Lipeurus caponis***

a – setae

Fig. 5 : ***Goniocotes gallinae***

a – eye, b – pronotum, c – seta

PLATE V

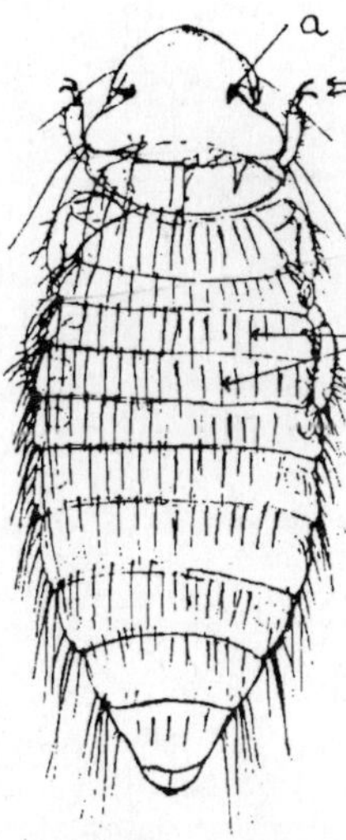

Fig. 1

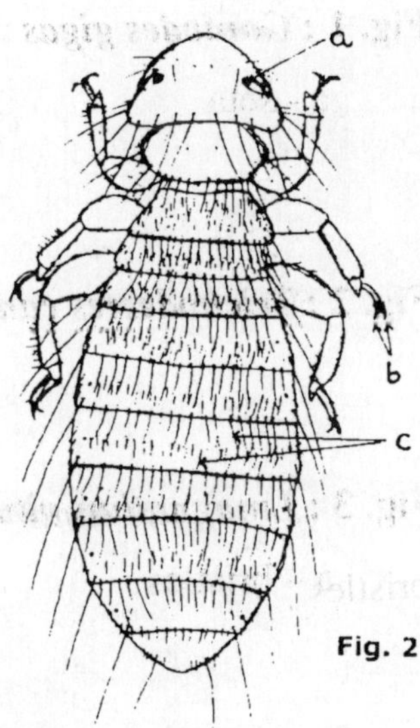

Fig. 2

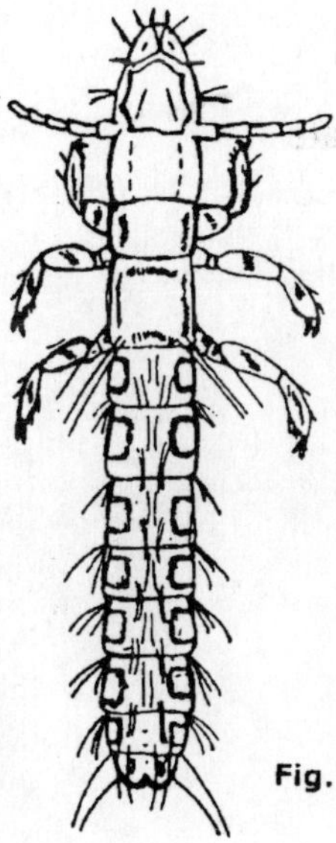

Fig. 3

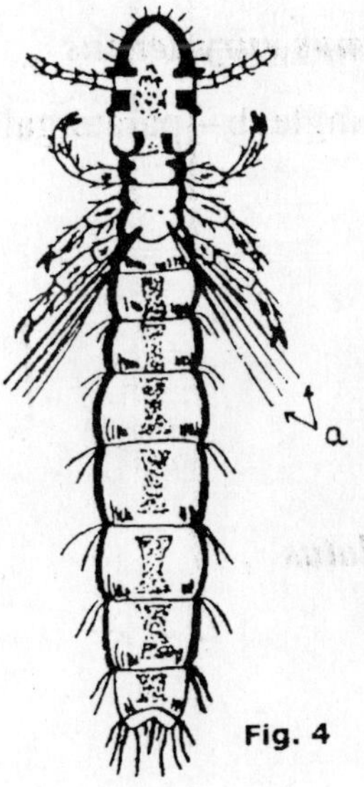

Fig. 4

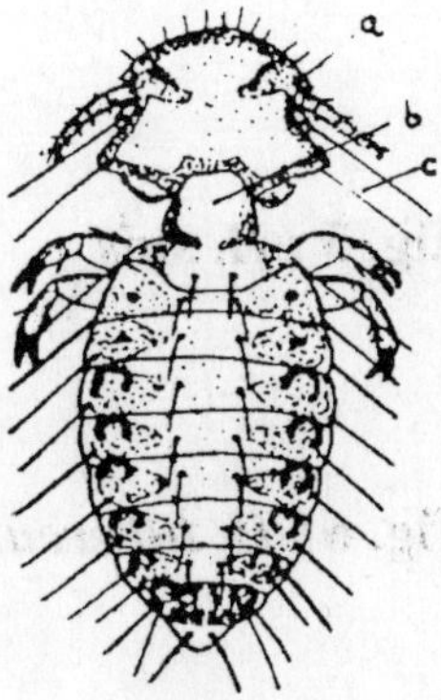

Fig. 5

PLATE VI

Fig. 1 : *Goniodes gigas*

a - seta

Fig. 2 : *Trichodectes canis*

Fig. 3 : *Linognathus vituli*

a – bristles

Fig. 4 : *Haematopinus eurysternus*

a – temporal angle, b – paratergal plate

Fig. 5 : *H. suis*

Fig. 6 : *H. tuberculatus*

PLATE VI

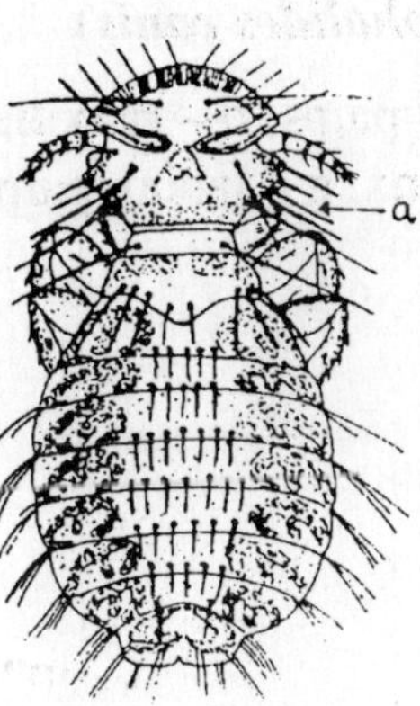

Fig. 1

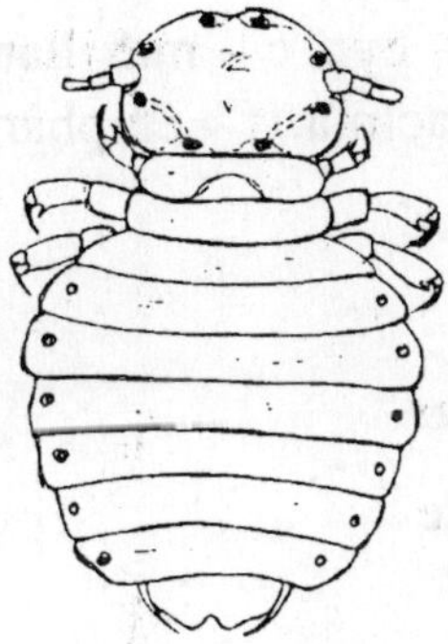

Fig. 2

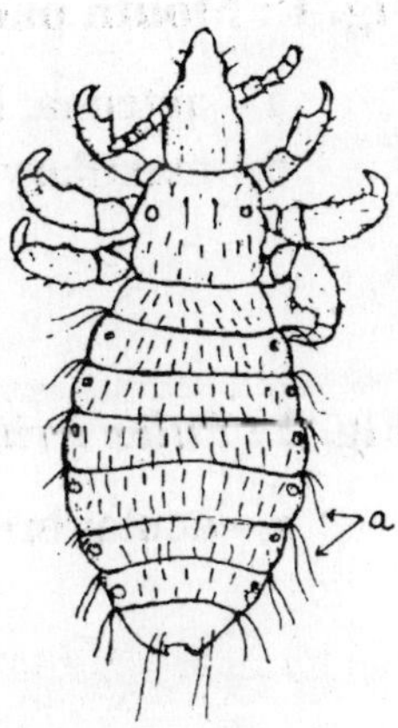

Fig. 3

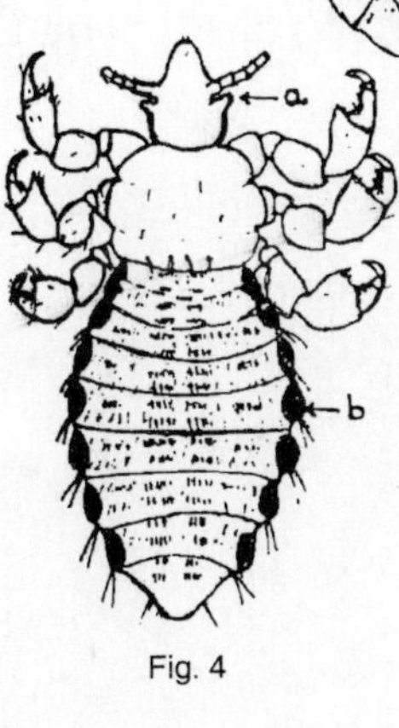

Fig. 4

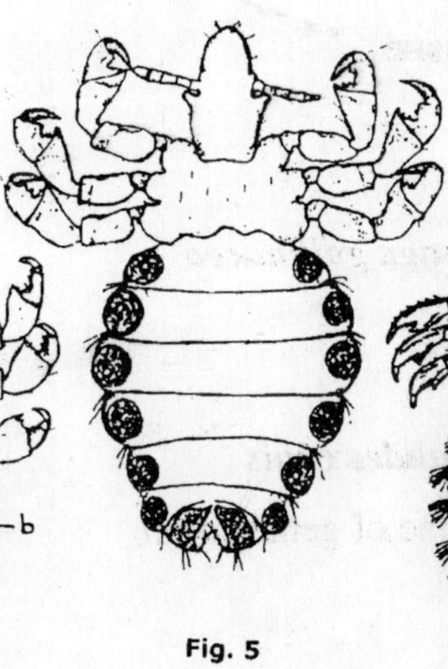

Fig. 5

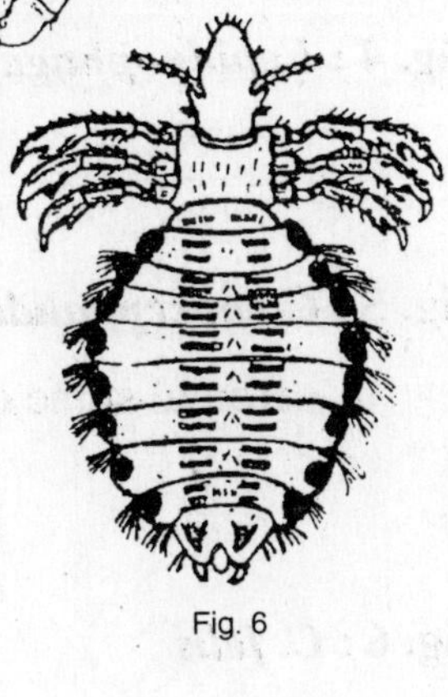

Fig. 6

PLATE VII

Fig. 1 : Mouth parts of a flea (*Ctenocephalides canis*)

a – antenna, b – eye, c – maxillary palps, d – maxillae, e – maxillary lacinia, f – epipharynx, g – labial palps

Fig. 2 : *Pulex irritans*

a – ocular bristle

Fig. 3 : *Xenopsylla cheopis*

a – ocular bristle

Fig. 4 : *Echidnophaga gallinacea*

Fig. 5 : *Ctenocephalides canis*

a – frontal spine of genal comb

Fig. 6 : *C. felis*

a – frontal spine of genal comb

PLATE VII

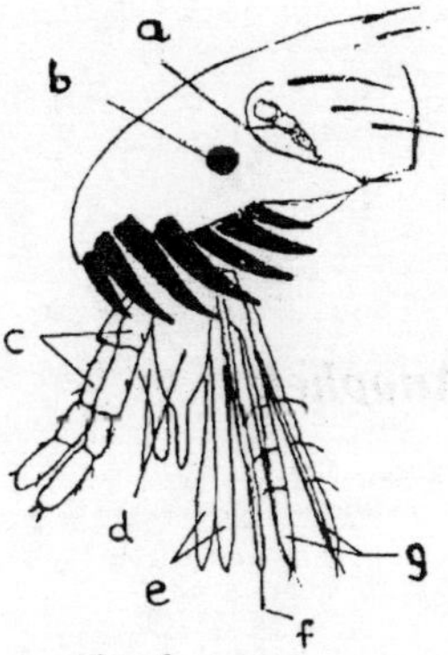

Fig. 1

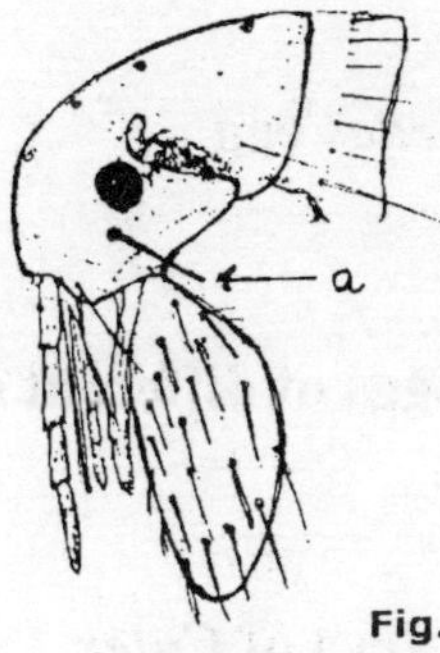

Fig. 2

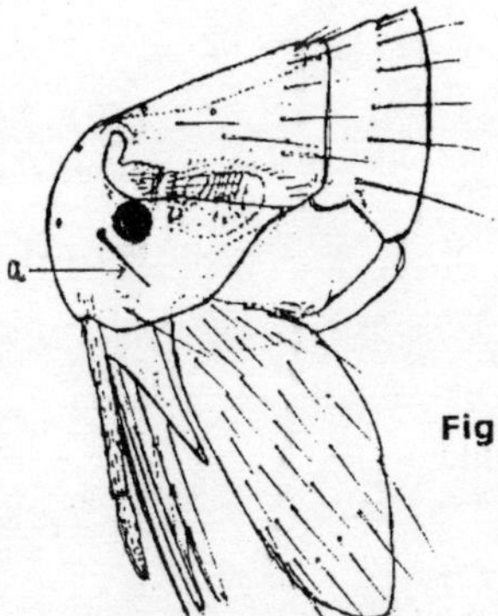

Fig. 3

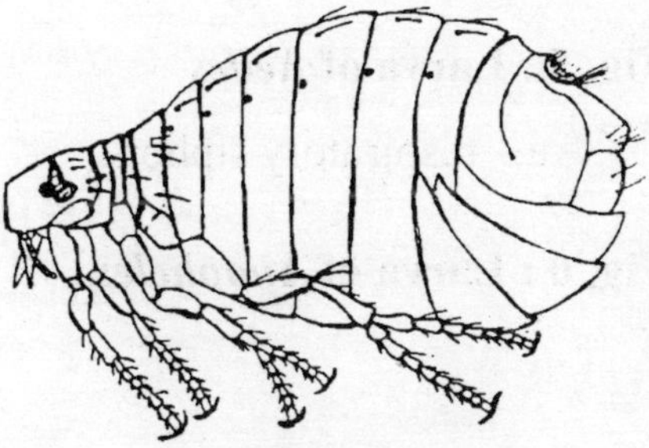

Fig. 4

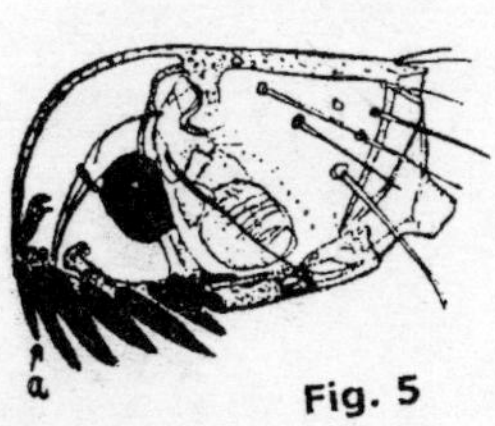

Fig. 5

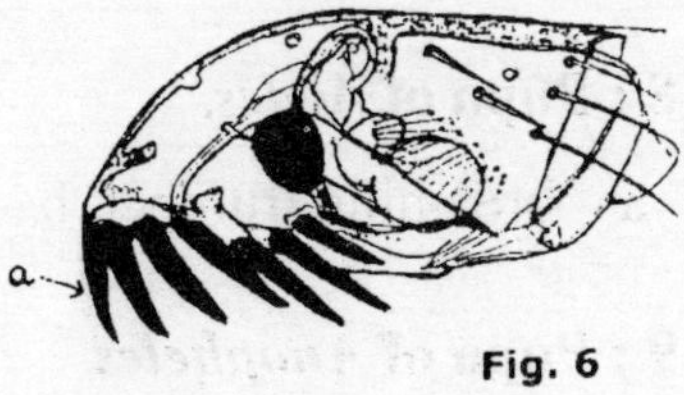

Fig. 6

PLATE VIII

Fig. 1 : Raft of *Culex* eggs

Fig. 2 : *Aedes* egg

Fig. 3 : Eggs of different species of *Anopheles*

Fig. 4 : Larva of *Culex*

a – respiratory siphon

Fig. 5 : Larva of *Aedes*

a – respiratory siphon

Fig. 6 : Larva of *Anopheles*

Fig. 7 : Pupa of *Culex*

a – breathing trumpet, b – paddle

Fig. 8 : Pupa of *Aedes*

a – breathing trumpet, b – paddle

Fig. 9 : Pupa of *Anopheles*

a – breathing trumpet, b – paddle

PLATE VIII

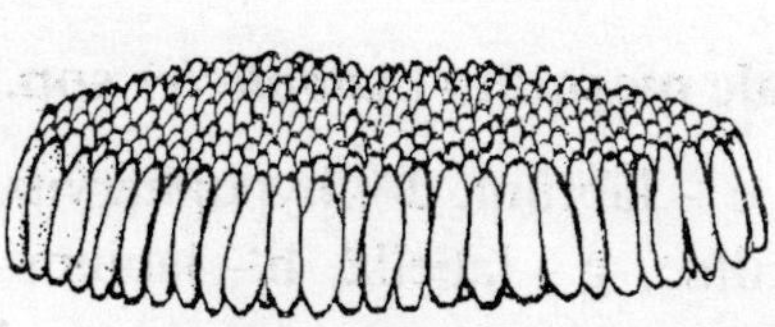

Fig. 1

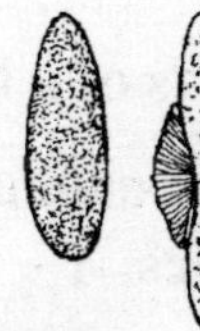

Fig. 2

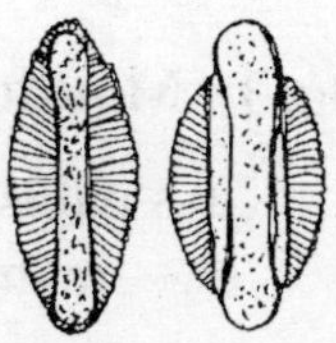

Fig. 3

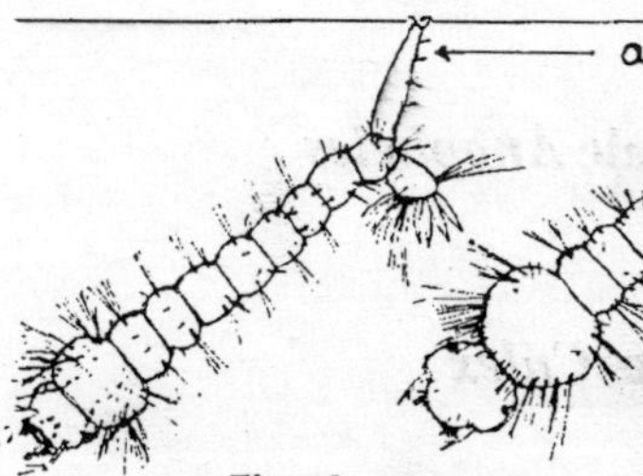

Fig. 4

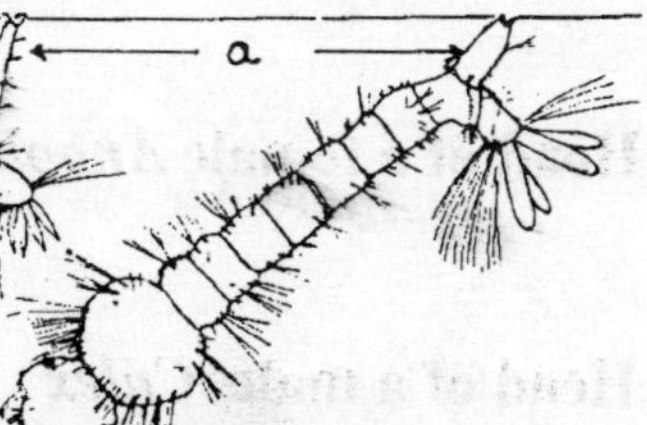

Fig. 5

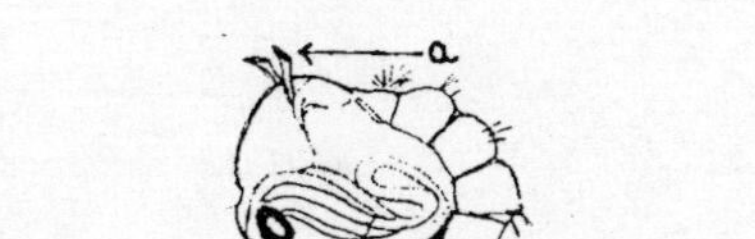

Fig. 6

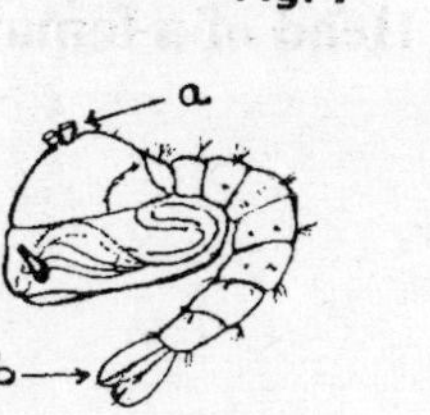

Fig. 7

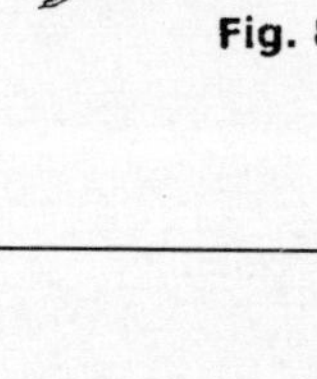

Fig. 8

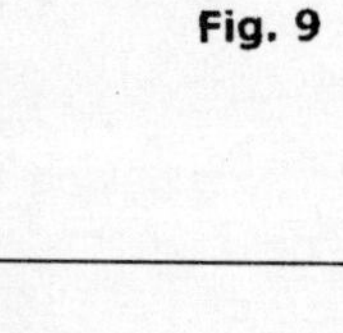

Fig. 9

PLATE IX

Fig. 1 : Mouthparts of a female mosquito (*Anopheles* spp.)

a – palps, b – antennae, c – labrum, d – hypopharynx, e – mandibles, f – maxillae, g – labella, h – labium

Fig. 2 : Head of a male *Anopheles*

Fig. 3 : Head of a female *Anopheles*

Fig. 4 : Head of a male *Culex*

Fig. 5 : Head of a female *Culex*

Fig. 6 : Head of a male *Aedes*

Fig. 7 : Head of a female *Aedes*

PLATE IX

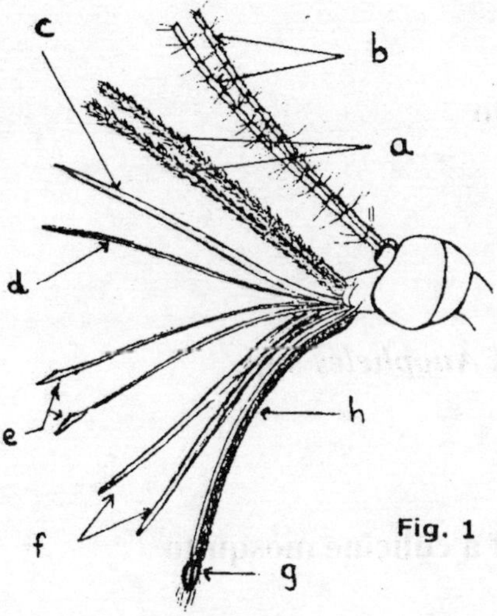

Fig. 1

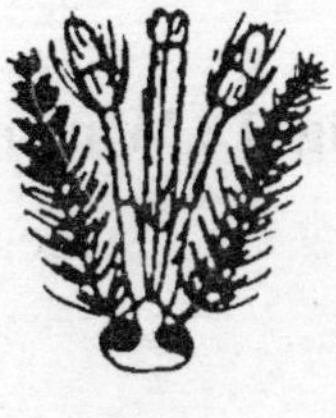

Fig. 2

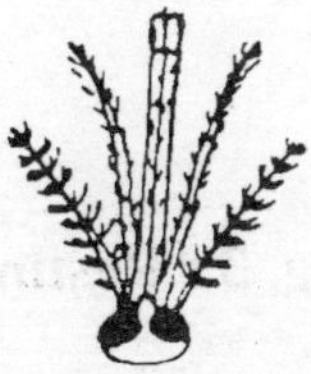

Fig. 3

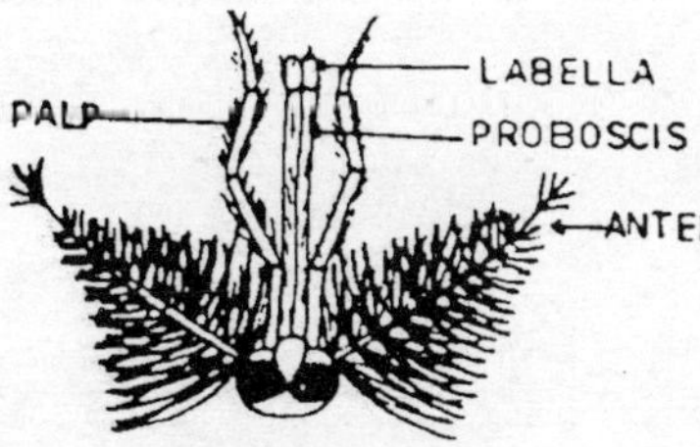

Fig. 4

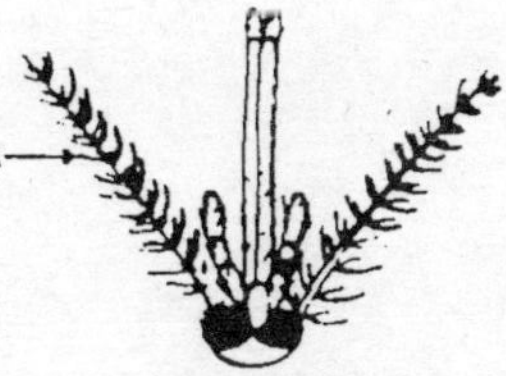

Fig. 5

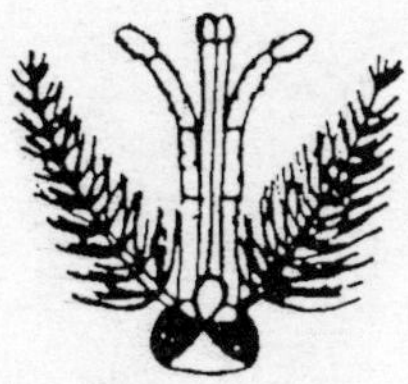

Fig. 6

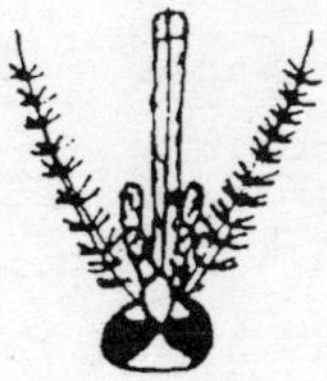

Fig. 7

PLATE X

Fig. 1 : Wing of a mosquito

a – scales

Fig. 2 : Resting position of *Anopheles* spp.

Fig. 3 : Resting position of a culicine mosquito

PLATE X

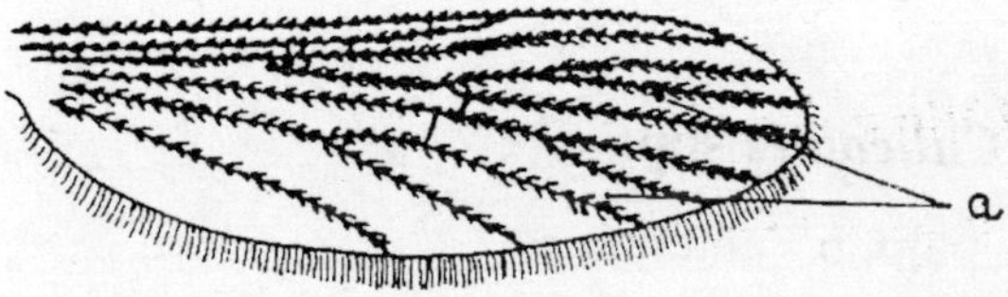

Fig. 1

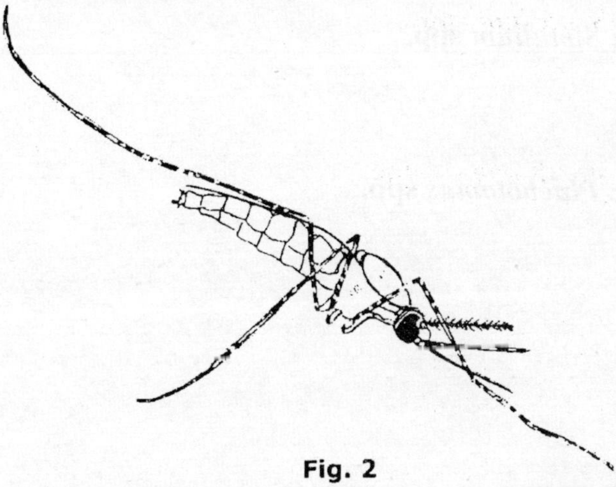

Fig. 2

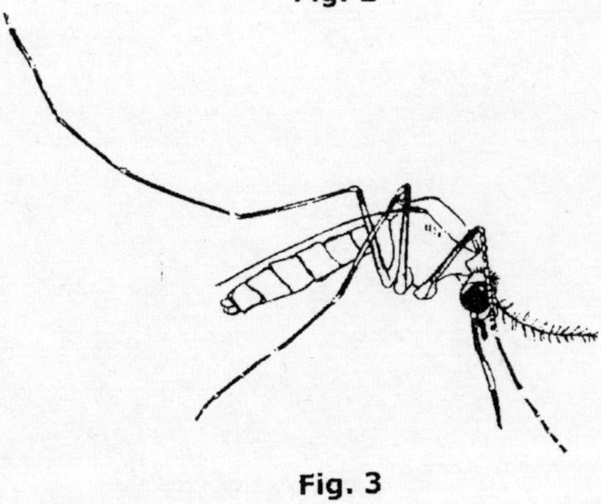

Fig. 3

PLATE XI

Fig. 1 : *Culicoides* spp.

a – palp, b - antenna

Fig. 2 : *Simulium* spp.

Fig. 3 : *Phlebotomus* spp.

PLATE XI

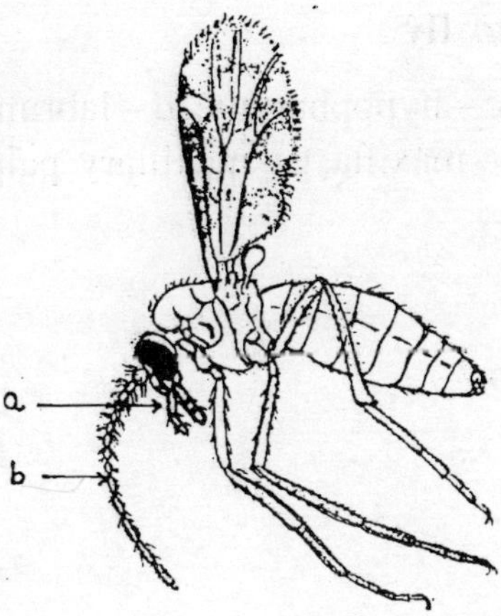

Fig. 1

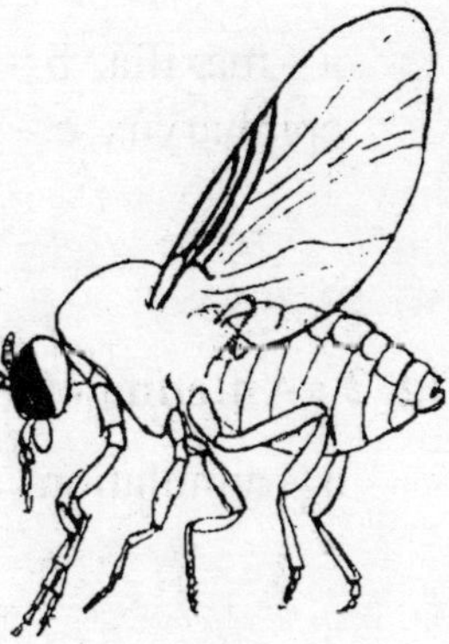

Fig. 2

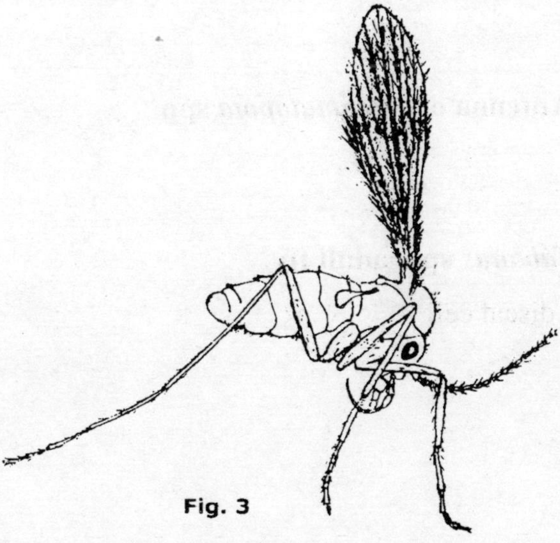

Fig. 3

PLATE XII

Fig. 1 : Mouthparts of a *Tabanus* fly

a – maxilla, b – mandible, c – hypopharynx, d – labrum epipharynx, e – mandible, f – maxilla, g – maxillary palp

Fig. 2 : Antenna of *Tabanus* spp.

a – annulations

Fig. 3 : Antenna of *Chrysops* spp.

Fig. 4 : Antenna of *Haematopota* spp.

Fig. 5 : *Tabanus* spp. adult fly

a – discal cell

PLATE XII

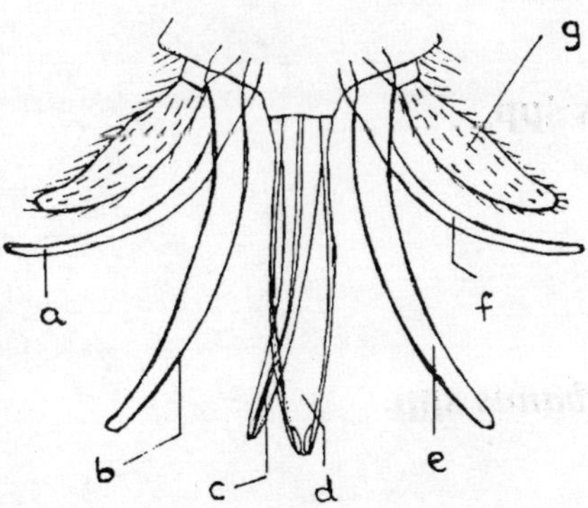

Fig. 1

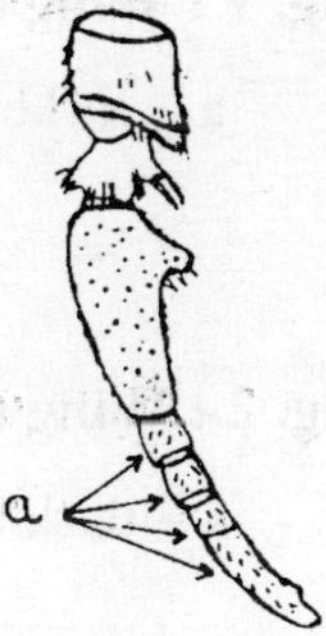

Fig. 2

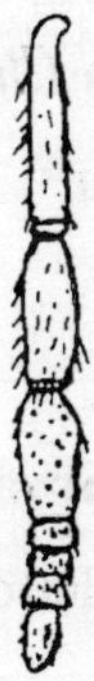

Fig. 3

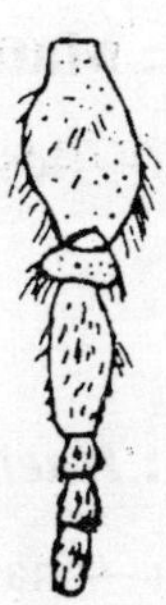

Fig. 4

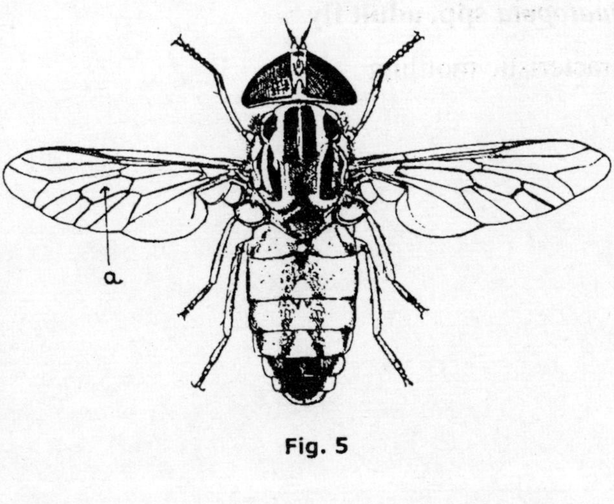

Fig. 5

PLATE XIII

Fig. 1 : Wing of a *Tabanus* spp.

a – forked vein near the tip, b – discal cell

Fig. 2 : Wing of a *Chrysops* spp.

a – dark band

Fig. 3 : Mature larva of *Tabanus* spp.

a – fleshy tubercles

Fig. 4 : *Haematopota* spp. adult fly

a – characteristic mottling

PLATE XIII

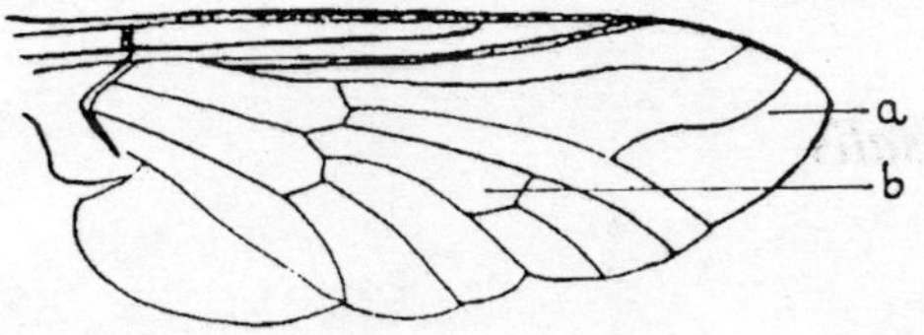

Fig. 1

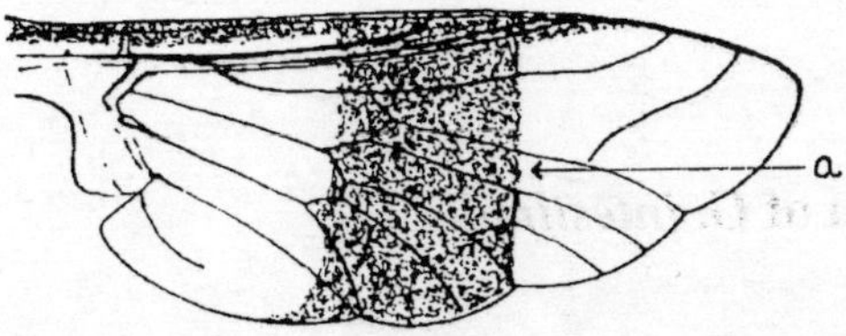

Fig. 2

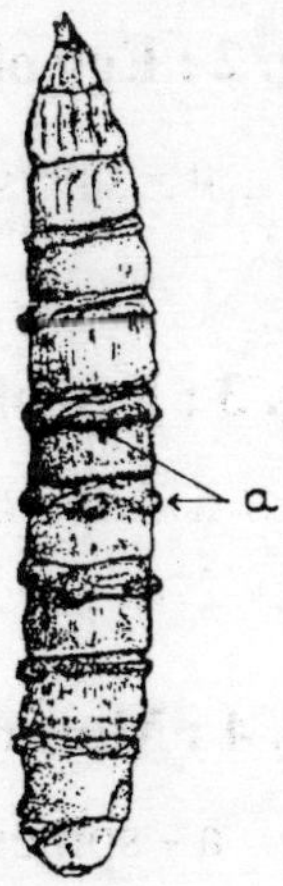

Fig. 3

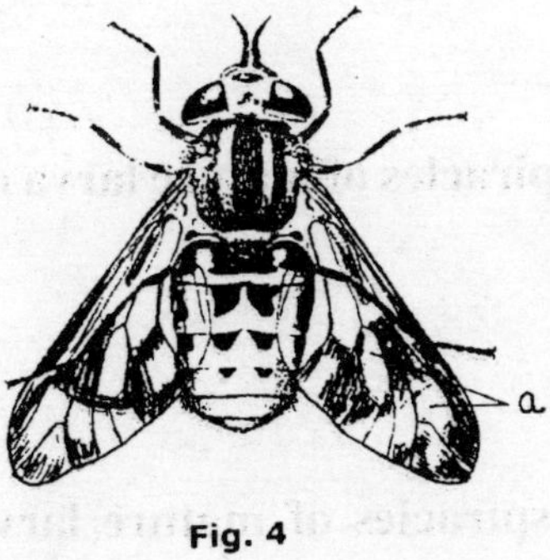

Fig. 4

PLATE XIV

Fig. 1 : *Gasterophilus* spp. adult fly

Fig. 2 : Egg of *G. nasalis*

a – operculum

Fig. 3 : Egg of *G. intestinalis*

a – operculum

Fig. 4 : Mature larva of *G. intestinalis*

a - spines

Fig. 5: Mature larva of *G. nasalis*

a - spines

Fig. 6: Posterior spiracles of mature larva of *Gasterophilus* spp.

a - slits

Fig. 7: Posterior spiracles of mature larva of *Cobboldia elephantis*

a - slits

PLATE XIV

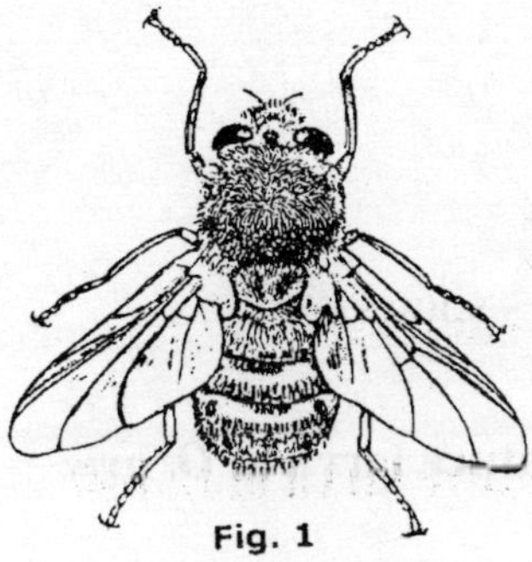

Fig. 1

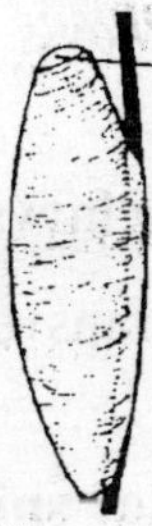

Fig. 2

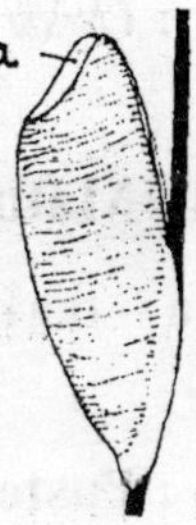

Fig. 3

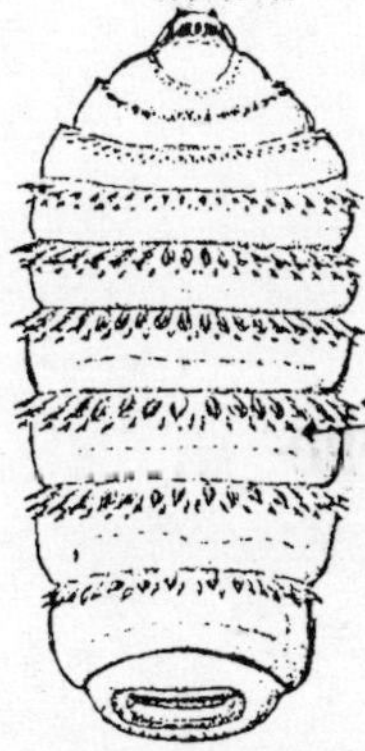

Fig. 4

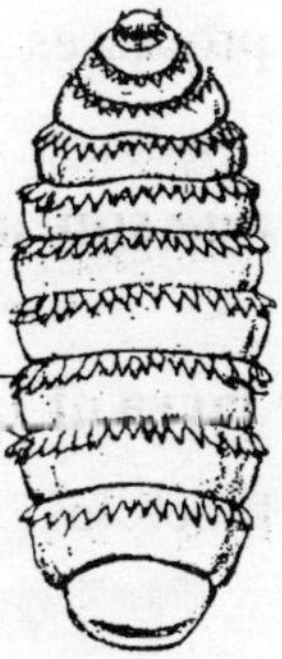

Fig. 5

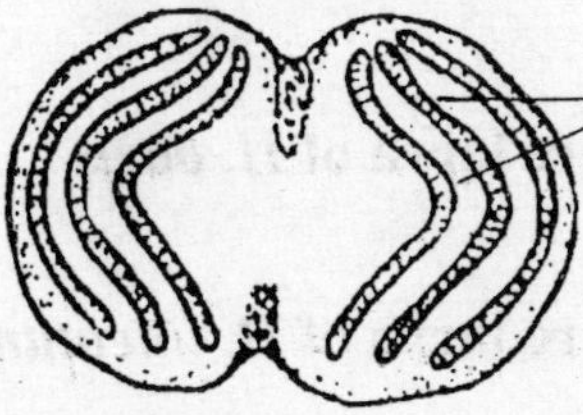

Fig. 6

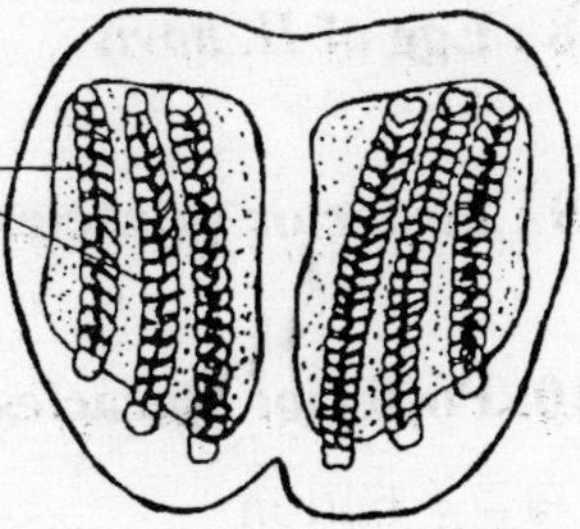

Fig. 7

PLATE XV

Fig. 1 : *Oestrus ovis* adult fly

Fig. 2 : Mature larva of *O. ovis*

a – dark transverse bands, b - spines

Fig. 3 : Posterior spiracles of mature larva of *O. ovis*

Fig. 4 : Mature larva of *Cephalopina titillator*

a – fleshy processes

Fig. 5 : *Hypoderma* spp. adult fly

Fig. 6 : Mature larva of *Hypoderma* spp.

a – fleshy tubercles

Fig. 7 : Eggs of *H. lineatum*

Fig. 8 : Egg of *H. bovis*

Fig. 9 : Posterior spiracles of mature larva of *H. bovis*

Fig.10: Posterior spiracles of mature larva of *H. lineatum*

a – button

PLATE XV

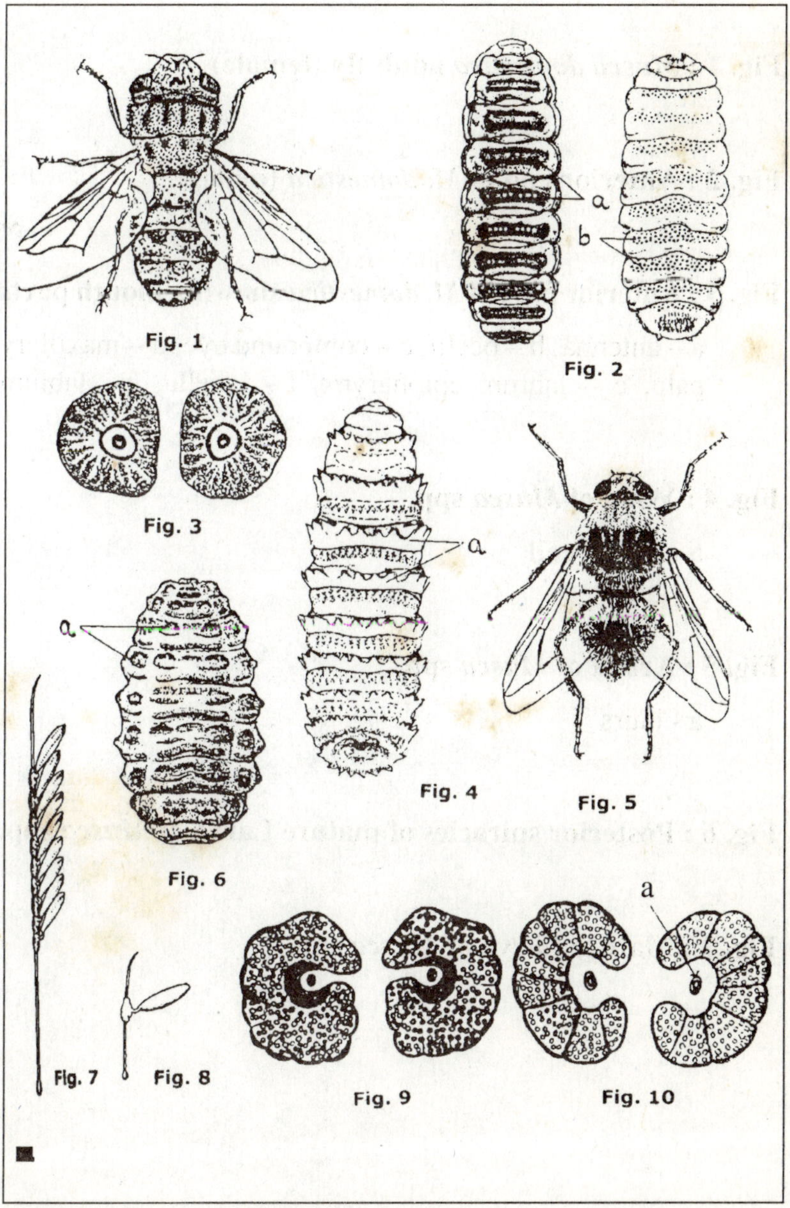

PLATE XVI

Fig. 1 : *Musca domestica* adult fly (female)

Fig. 2 : Anterior end of *M. domestica* (male)

Fig. 3 : Anterior part of *M. domestica* showing mouth parts

a – antenna, b – ocelli, c – compound eye, d – maxillary palp, e – labrum epipharynx, f – labella, g – labium

Fig. 4 : Wing of *Musca* spp.

a – apical cell

Fig. 5 : Arista of *Musca* spp.

a - hairs

Fig. 6 : Posterior spiracles of mature Larva of *Musca* spp.

Fig. 7 : Mature Larva of *Musca* spp.

PLATE XVI

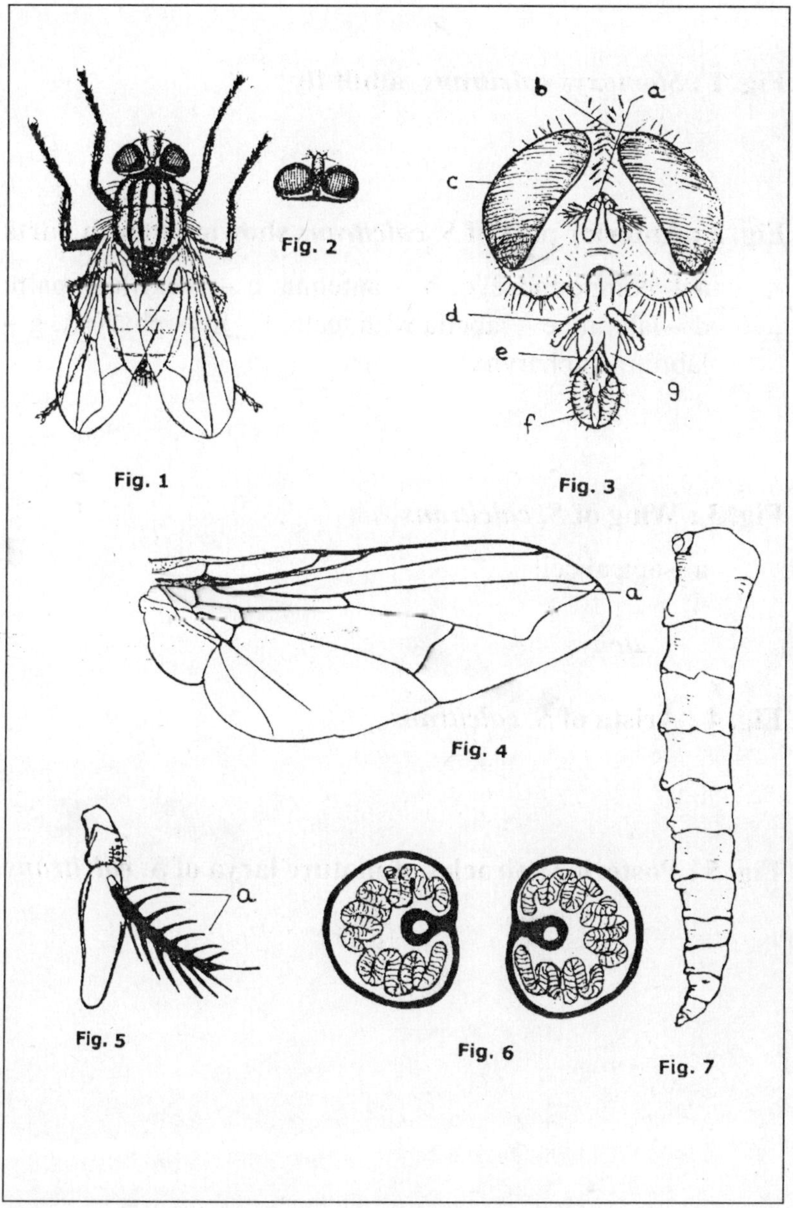

PLATE XVII

Fig. 1 : *Stomoxys calcitrans* adult fly

Fig. 2 : Anterior part of *S. calcitrans* showing mouth parts

a – compound eye, b – antenna, c – maxillary palp, d – labium, e – labella with teeth, f – hypopharynx, g – labrum epipharynx

Fig. 3 : Wing of *S. calcitrans*

a – apical cell

Fig. 4 : Arista of *S. calcitrans*

Fig. 5 : Posterior spiracles of mature larva of *S. calcitrans*

PLATE XVII

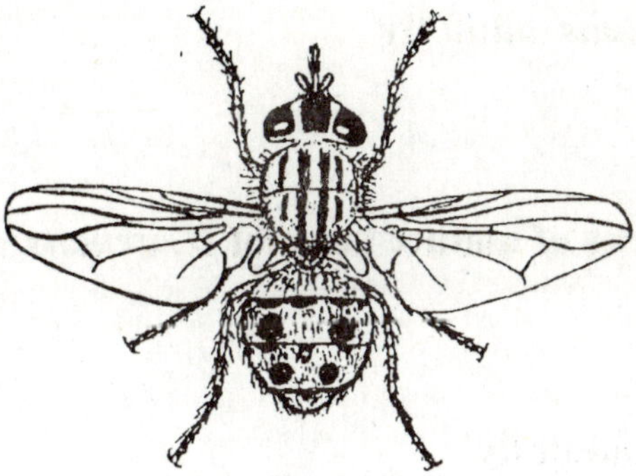

Fig. 1

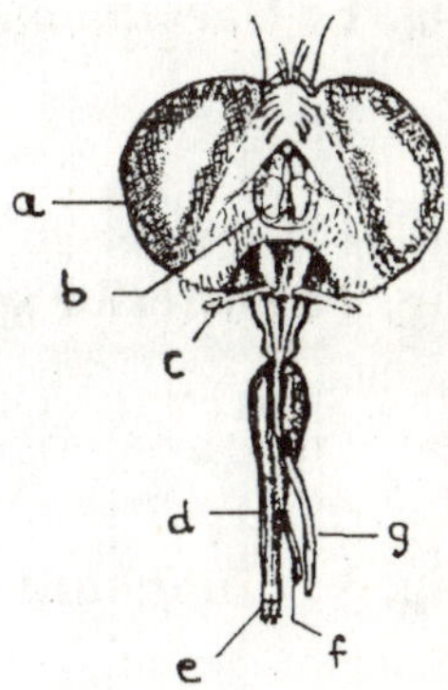

Fig. 2

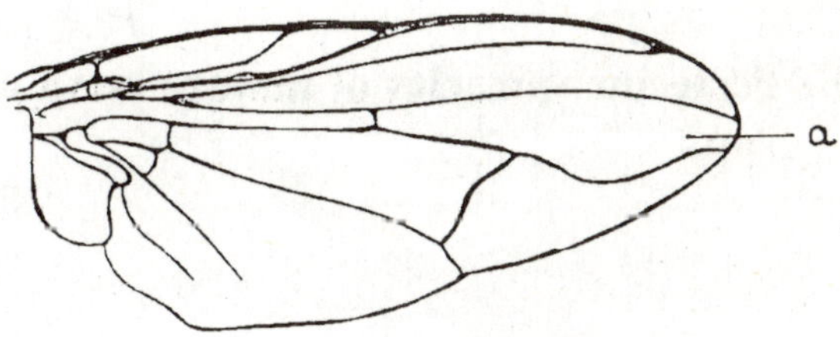

Fig. 3

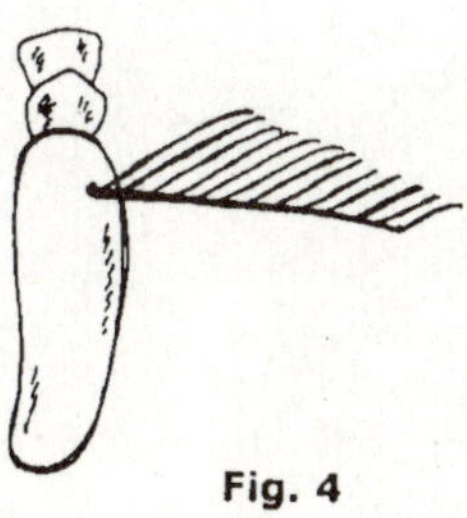

Fig. 4

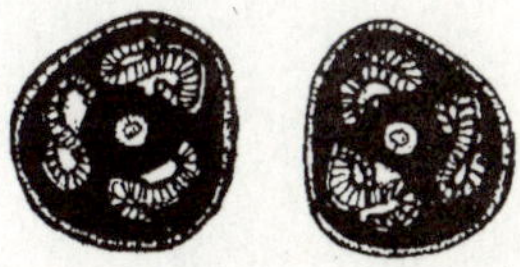

Fig. 5

PLATE XVIII

Fig. 1 : *Haematobia irritans* adult fly

Fig. 2 : Posterior spiracles of mature larva of *H. irritans*

Fig. 3 : *Calliphora* spp. adult fly

Fig. 4 : Posterior spiracles of mature larva of *Calliphora* spp.

Fig. 5 : Mature larva of *Calliphora* spp.

PLATE XVIII

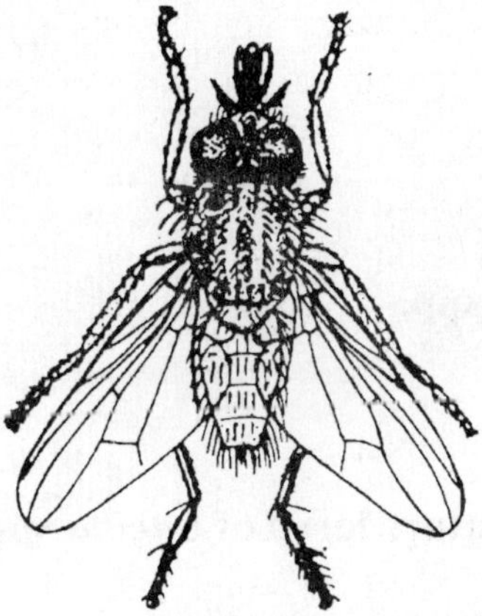

Fig. 1

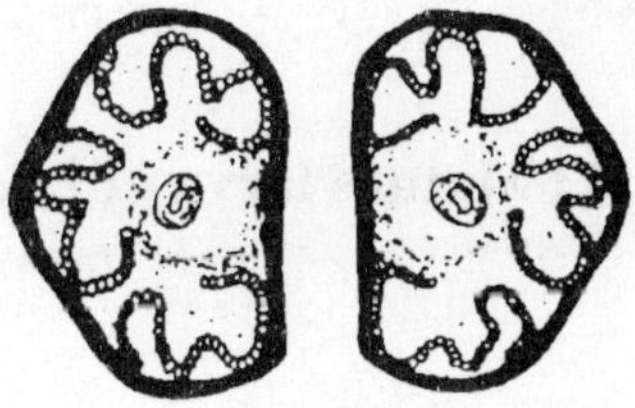

Fig. 2

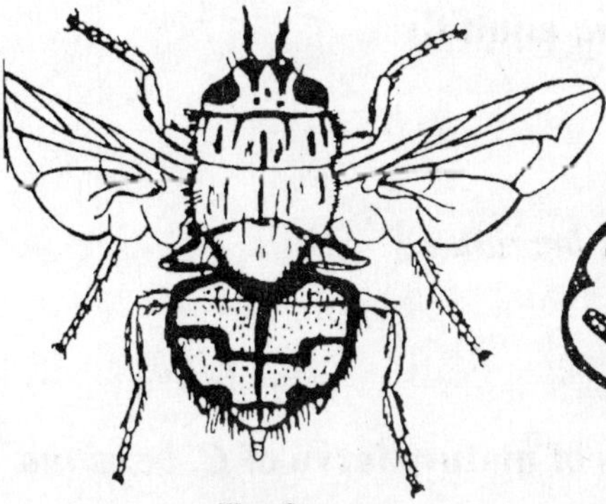

Fig. 3

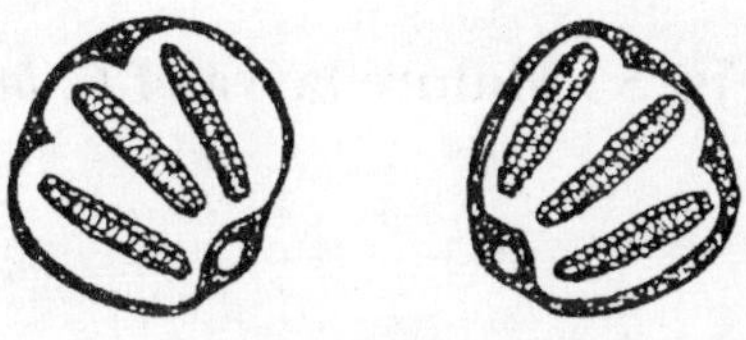

Fig. 4

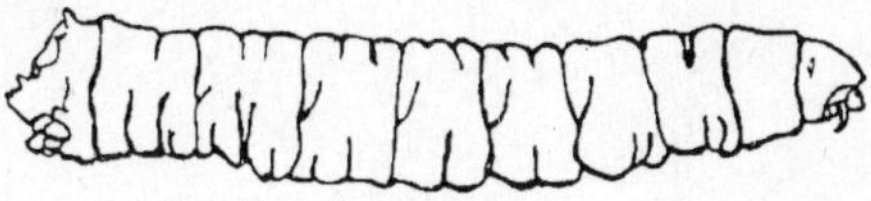

Fig. 5

PLATE XIX

Fig. 1 : *Lucilia* spp. adult fly

Fig. 2 : Mature larva of *Lucilia* spp.

Fig. 3 : Posterior spiracles of mature larva of *Lucilia* spp.

Fig. 4 : *Chrysomya bezziana* adult fly

Fig. 5 : Mature larva of *C. bezziana*

Fig. 6 : Posterior spiracles of mature larva of *C. bezziana*

PLATE XIX

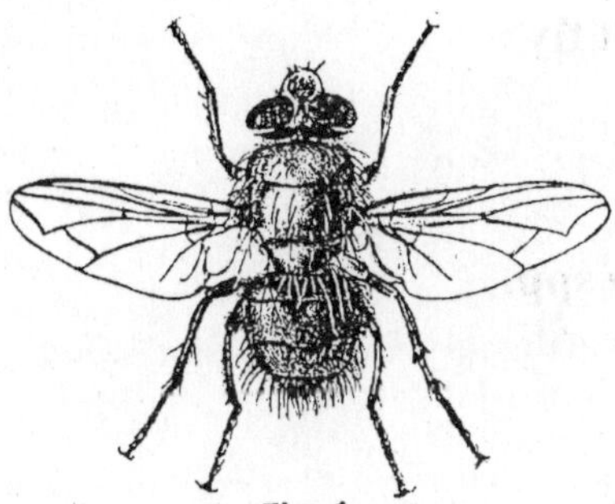

Fig. 1

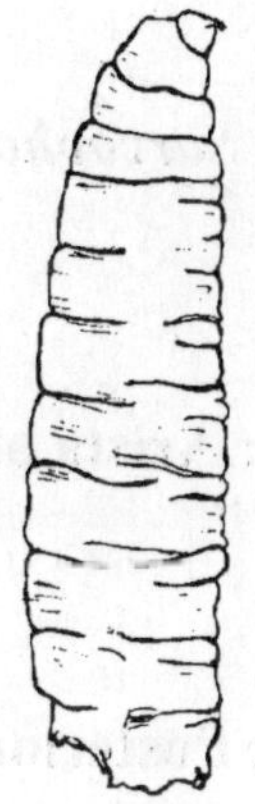

Fig. 2

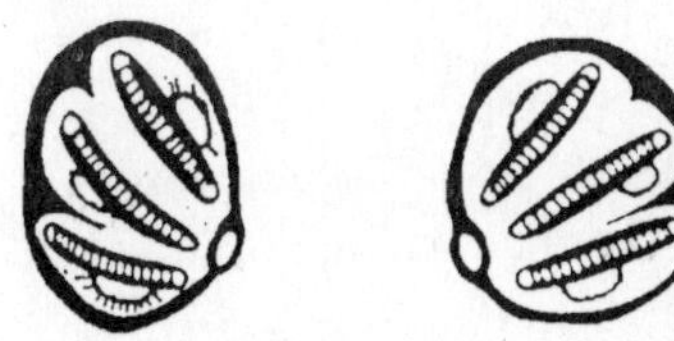

Fig. 3

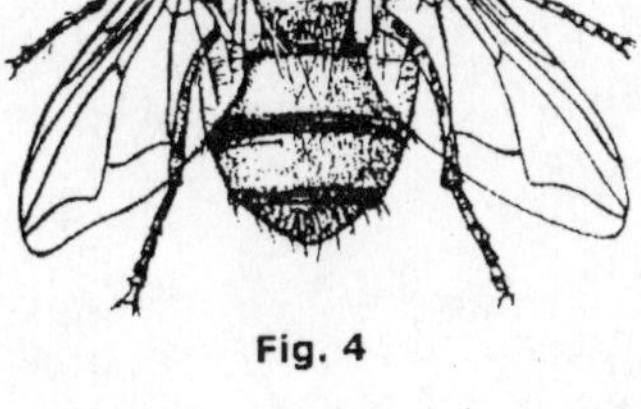

Fig. 4

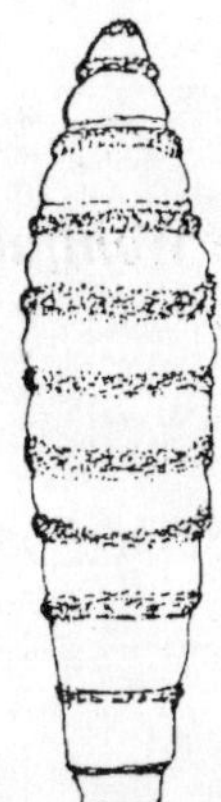

Fig. 5

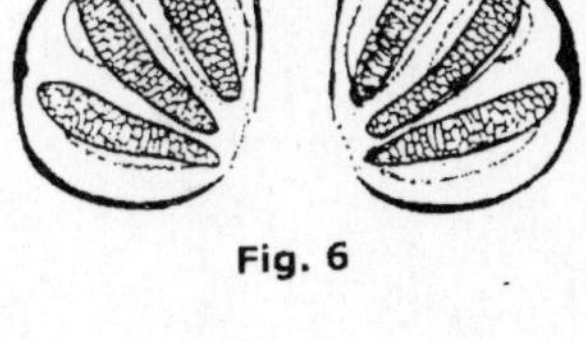

Fig. 6

PLATE XX

Fig. 1 : *Sarcophaga* spp. adult fly

Fig. 2 : Arista of *Sarcophaga* spp.

Fig. 3 : Posterior spiracles of mature larva of *Sarcophaga* spp.

Fig. 4 : *Wohlfahrtia* spp. adult fly

PLATE XX

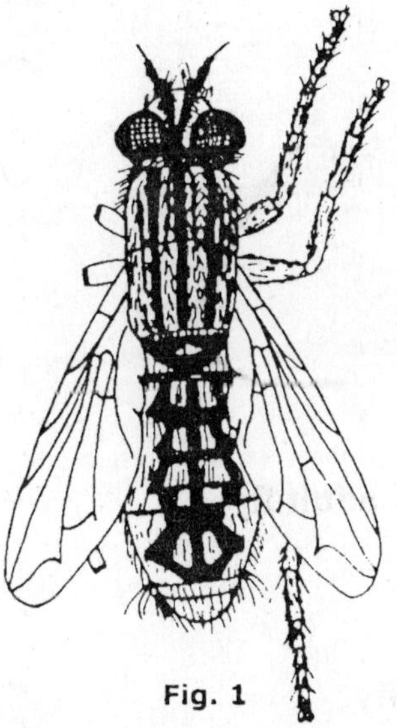

Fig. 1

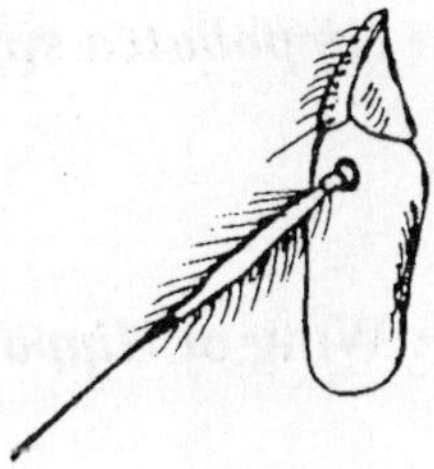

Fig. 2

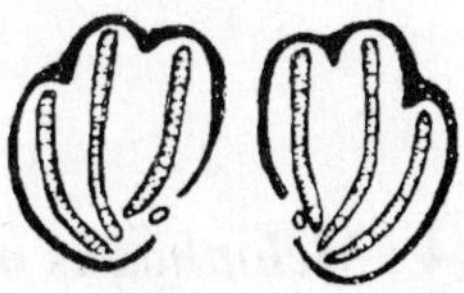

Fig. 3

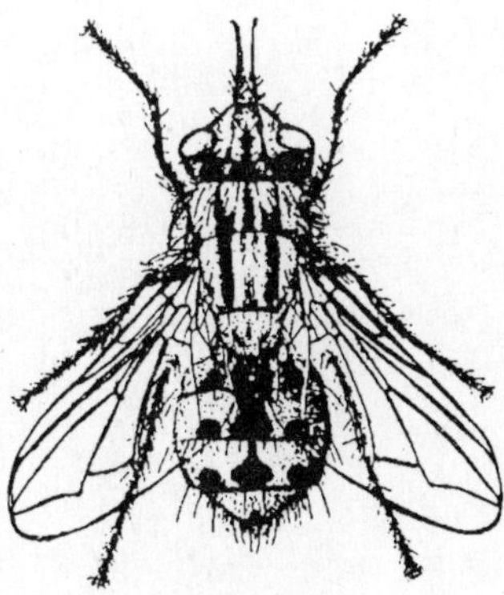

Fig. 4

PLATE XXI

Fig. 1 : *Hippobosca* spp. adult fly

Fig. 2 : Wing of *Hippobosca* spp.

Fig. 3 : *Pseudolynchia canariensis* adult fly

Fig. 4 : *Melophagus ovinus* adult fly

PLATE XXI

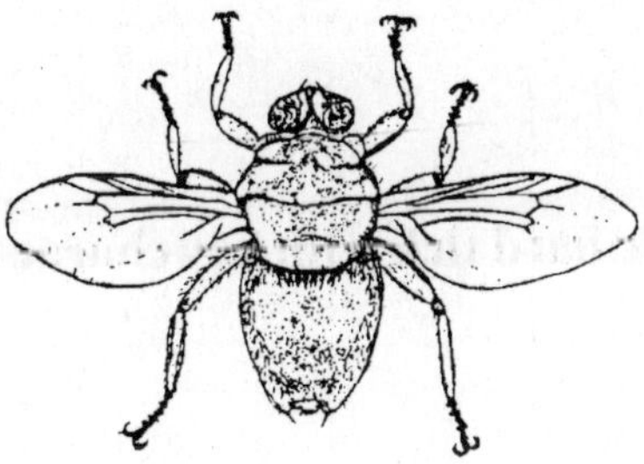

Fig. 1

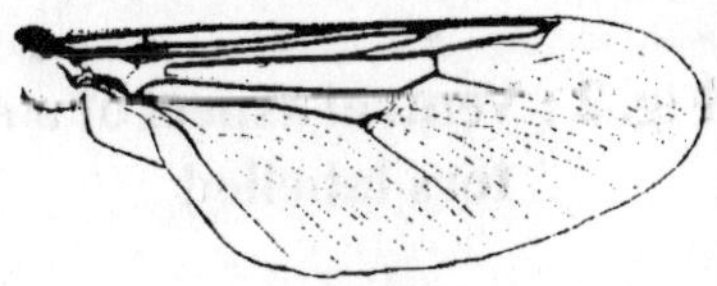

Fig. 2

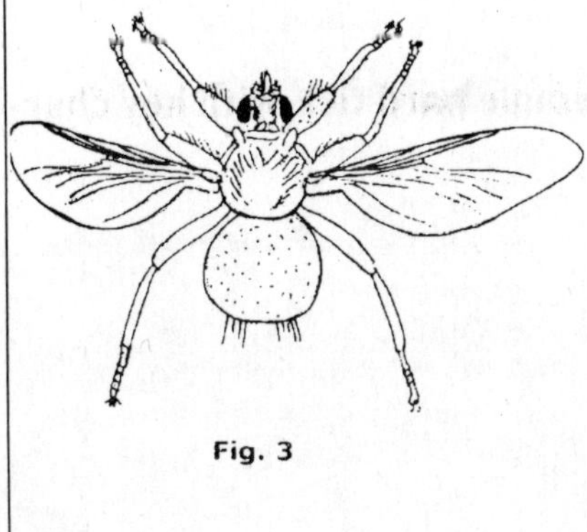

Fig. 3

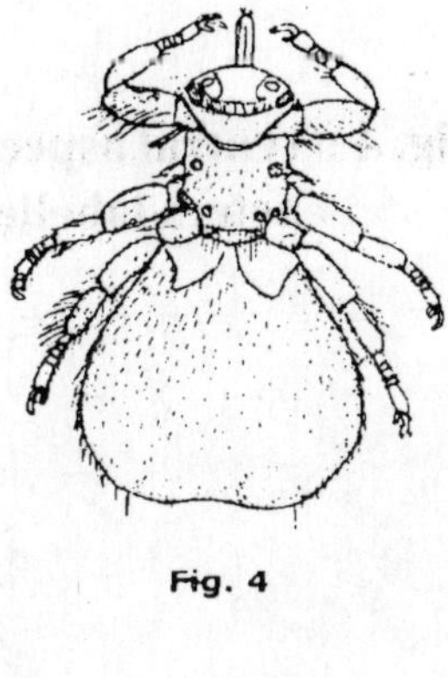

Fig. 4

PLATE XXII

Fig. 1 : Dorsal aspect of a male hard tick with key characters labelled

Fig. 2 : Ventral aspect of a male hard tick with key characters labelled

Fig. 3 : Dorsal aspect of a female hard tick with key characters labelled

Fig. 4 : Ventral aspect of a female hard tick with key characters labelled

PLATE XXII

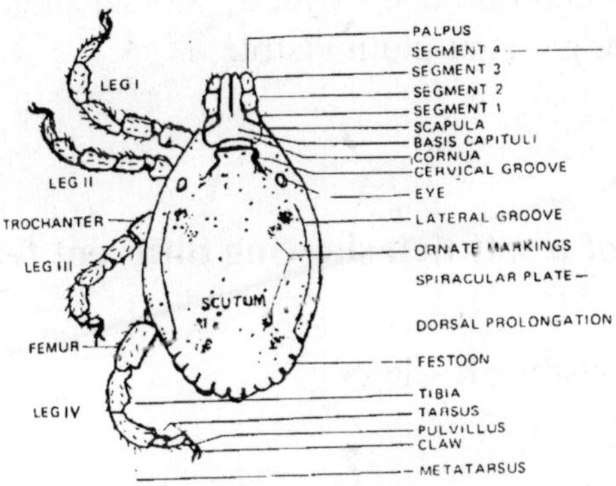

Fig. 1

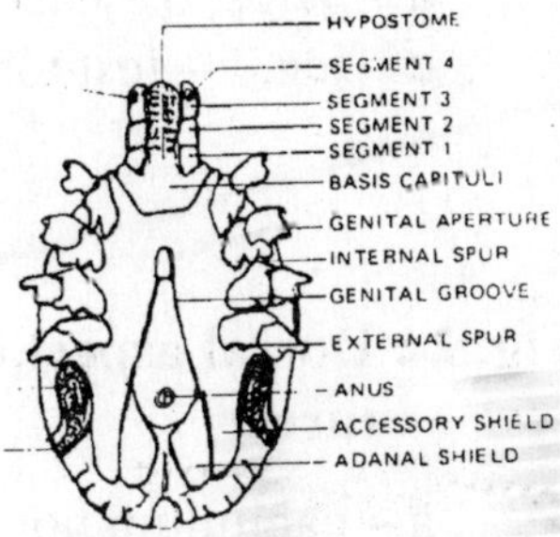

Fig. 2

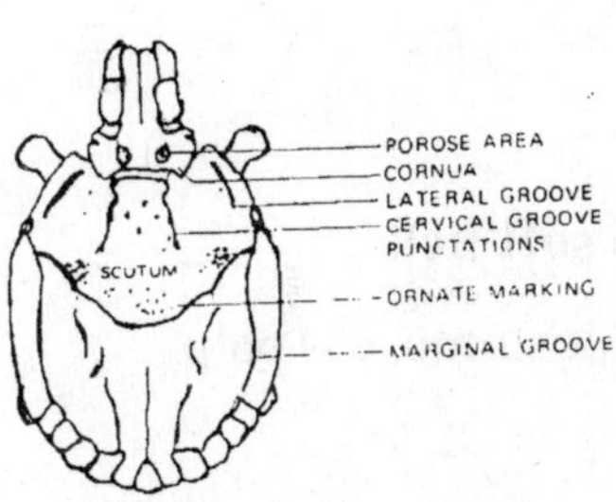

Fig. 3

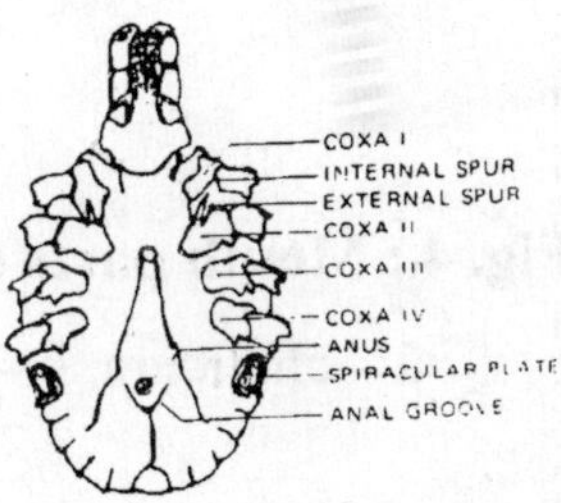

Fig. 4

PLATE XXIII

Fig. 1 : Dorsal aspect of a female hard tick showing different features

a – palps, b – basis capitulum, c – eye, d – dorsal shield, e – leg, f – festoon, g – capitulum visible

Fig. 2 : Dorsal aspect of a soft tick showing different features

a – capitulum not visible, b – leg

Fig. 3 : Mouth parts of a hard tick

a – chelicerae, b – cheliceral sheath, c – hypostome, d – basis capitulum, e – palp

Fig. 4 : Mouth parts of a soft tick

a – chelicera, b – hypostome, c – palp

PLATE XXIII

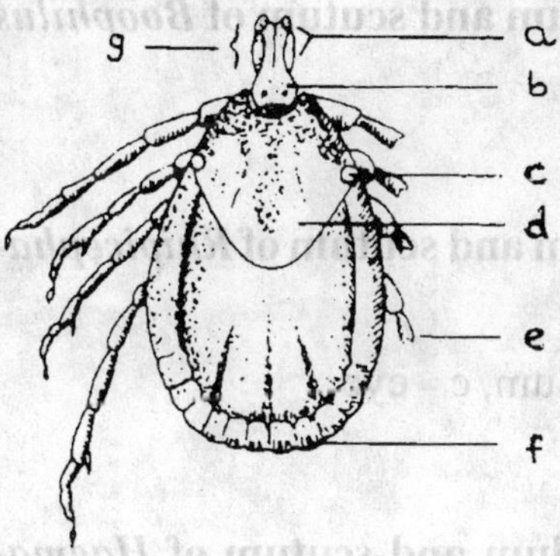

Fig. 1

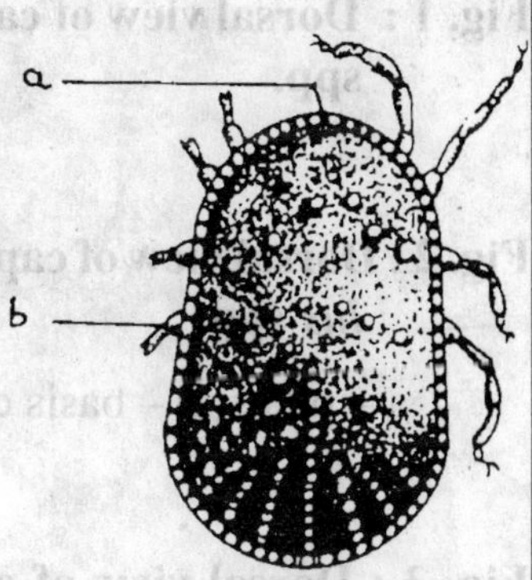

Fig. 2

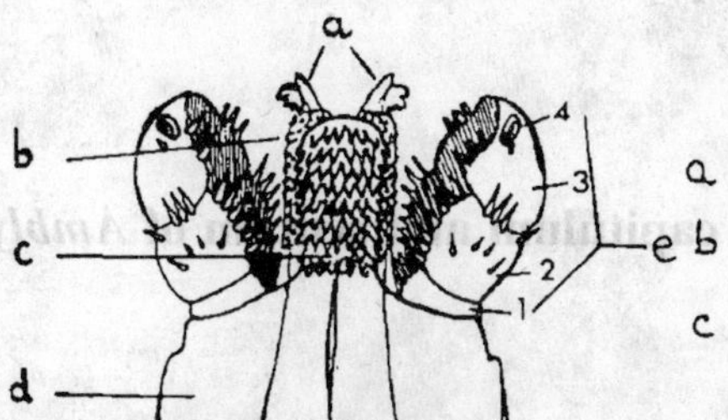

Fig. 3

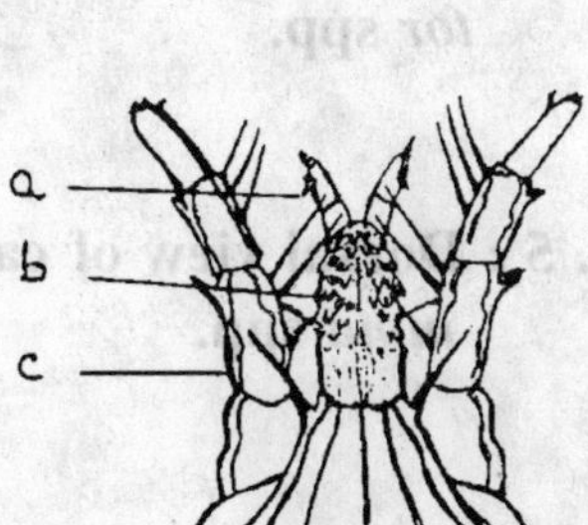

Fig. 4

PLATE XXIV

Fig. 1 : Dorsal view of capitulum and scutum of *Boophilus* spp.

Fig. 2 : Dorsal view of capitulum and scutum of *Rhipicephalus* spp.

a – palps, b – basis capitulum, c - eye

Fig. 3 : Dorsal view of capitulum and scutum of *Haemaphysalis* spp.

a – porose area

Fig. 4 : Dorsal view of capitulum and scutum of *Dermacentor* spp.

Fig. 5 : Dorsal view of capitulum and scutum of *Amblyomma* spp.

Fig. 6 : Dorsal view of capitulum and scutum of *Ixodes* spp.

PLATE XXIV

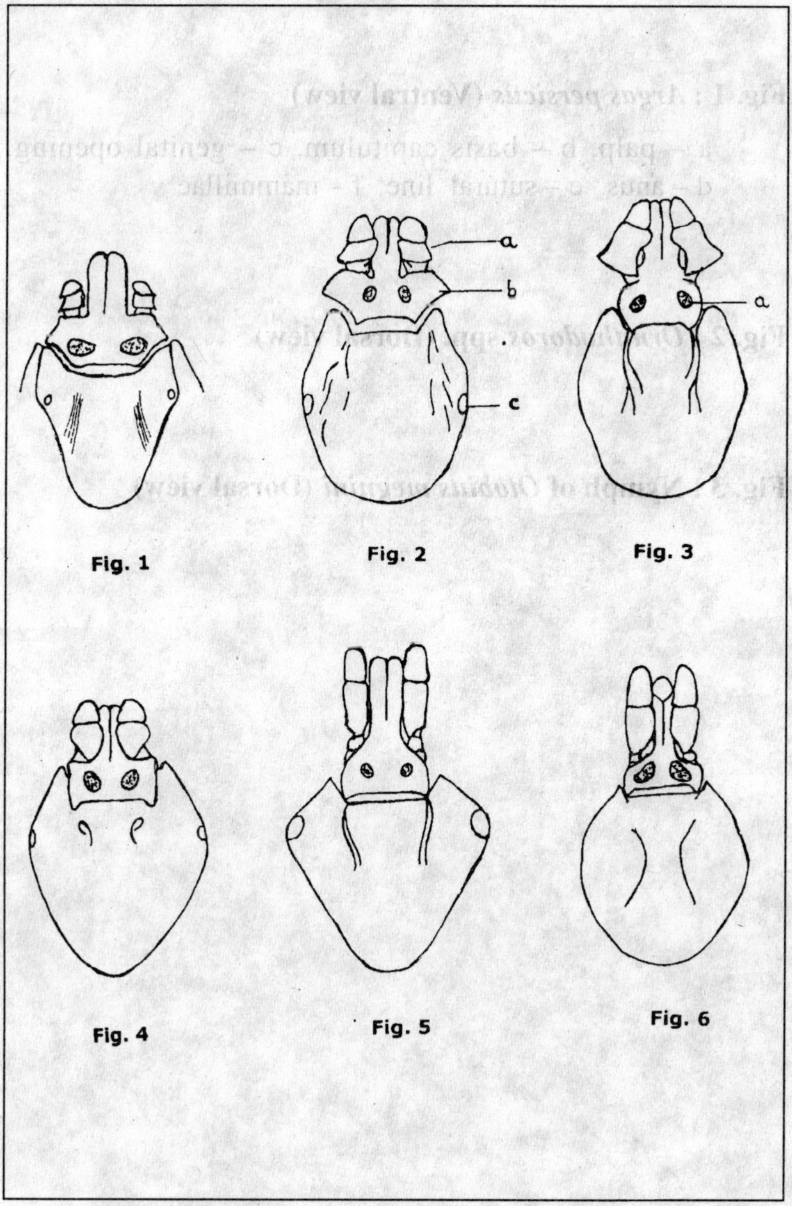

PLATE XXV

Fig. 1 : *Argas persicus* (Ventral view)

a – palp, b – basis capitulum, c – genital opening, d – anus, e – sutural line, f – mammillae

Fig. 2 : *Ornithodoros* spp. (Dorsal view)

Fig. 3 : Nymph of *Otobius megnini* (Dorsal view)

PLATE XXV

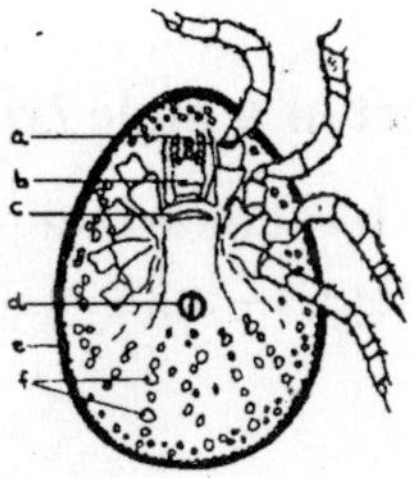

Fig. 1

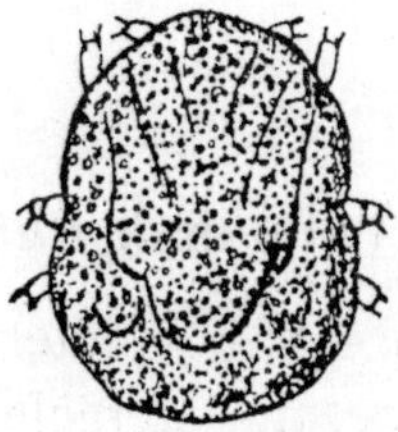

Fig. 2

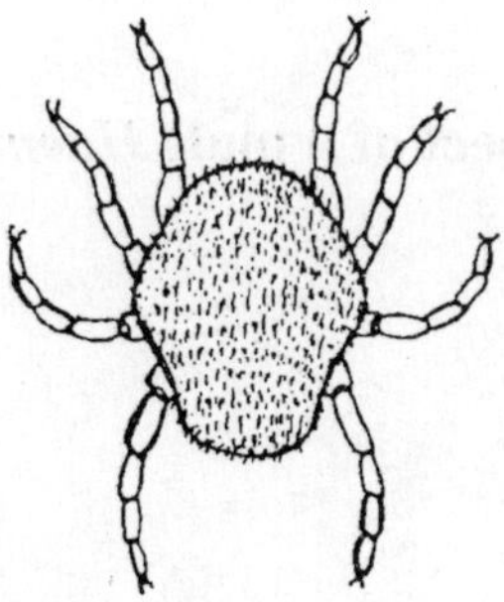

Fig. 3

PLATE XXVI

Fig. 1 : Ventral aspect of a male *Ixodes* spp.

a – capitulum, b – coxa-I, c – coxal spur, d – adanal plate, e – anal plate, f – anus, g – median plate, h – genital orifice

Fig. 2 : Ventral aspect of a male *Boophilus microplus*

Fig. 3 : Ventral aspect of a male *Rhipicephalus* spp.

a – palpal article -IV, b – internal and external spurs, c – genital orifice, d – spiracle, e – accessory shield, f – anal groove, g – festoons, h – postanal median groove, i – adanal shield, j - anus

Fig. 4 : Ventral aspect of a male *Haemaphysalis* spp.

PLATE XXVI

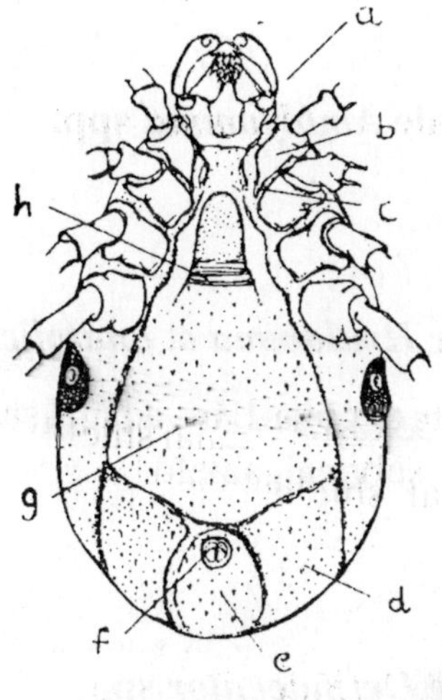

Fig. 1

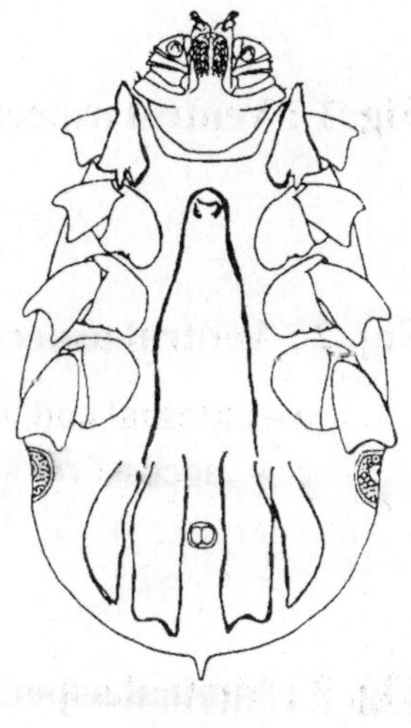

Fig. 2

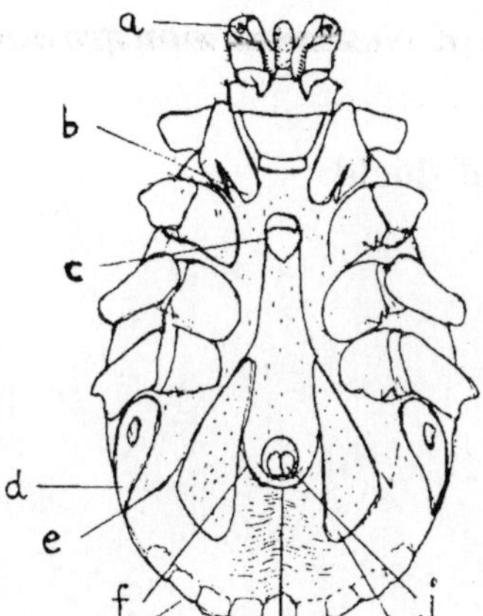

Fig. 3

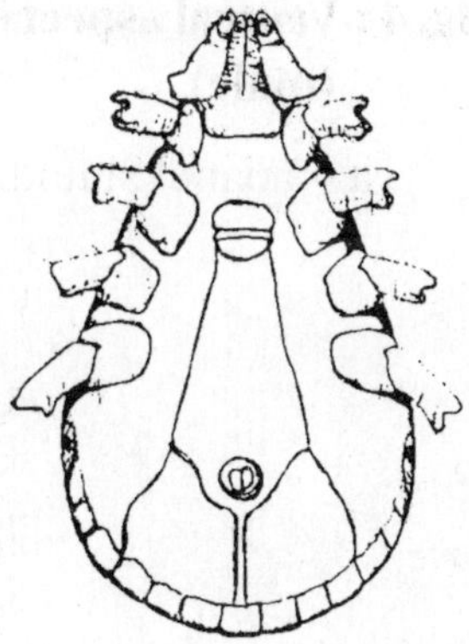

Fig. 4

PLATE XXVII

Fig. 1 : Ventral aspect of a female *Amblyomma* spp.

Fig. 2 : Ventral aspect of a male *Hyalomma a. anatolicum*

a – external and internal spurs of coxa-I, b – adanal shield, c – accessory shield, d – subanal shield

Fig. 3 : Ventral aspect of a male *Dermacentor* spp.

Fig. 4 : Ventral aspect of idiosoma of *Nosomma monstrosum* (male)

a – adanal shield, b – subanal shield

PLATE XXVII

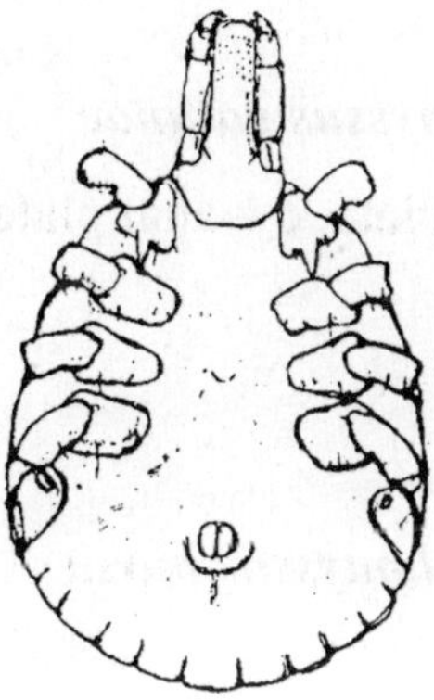

Fig. 1

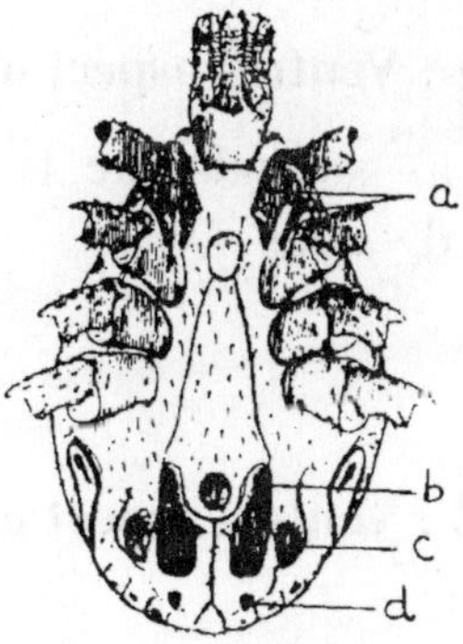

Fig. 2

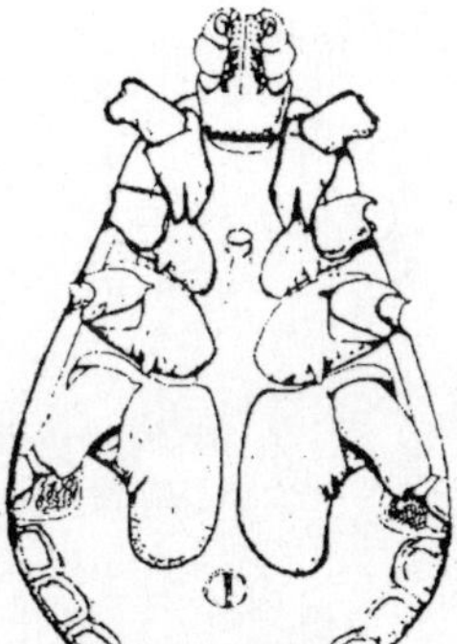

Fig. 3

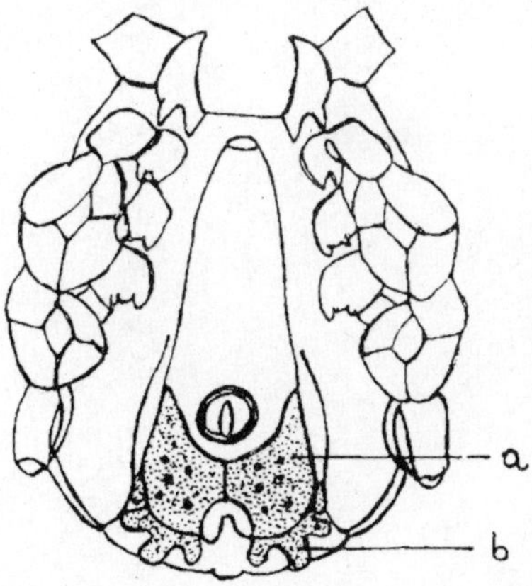

Fig. 4

PLATE XXVIII

Fig. 1 : Ventral aspect of a male *Dermanyssus gallinae*

a – sternal plate, b – genito-ventral plate, c – anal plate, d – anus

Fig. 2 : Ventral aspect of a female *Ornithonyssus bursa*

Fig. 3 : Ventral aspect of a female *Sarcoptes scabiei*

Fig. 4 : Dorsal aspect of a female *Cnemidocoptes mutans*

PLATE XXVIII

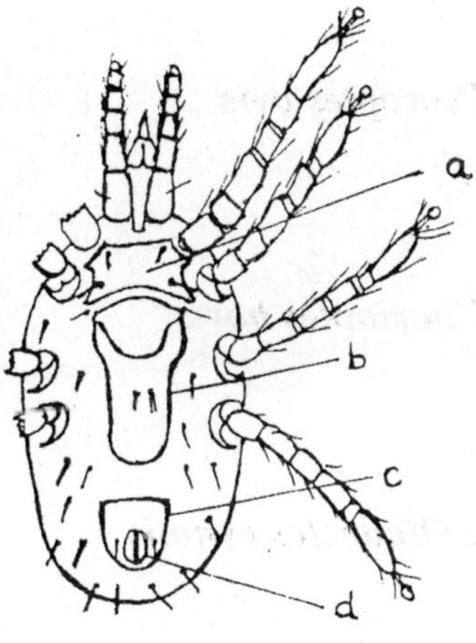

Fig. 1

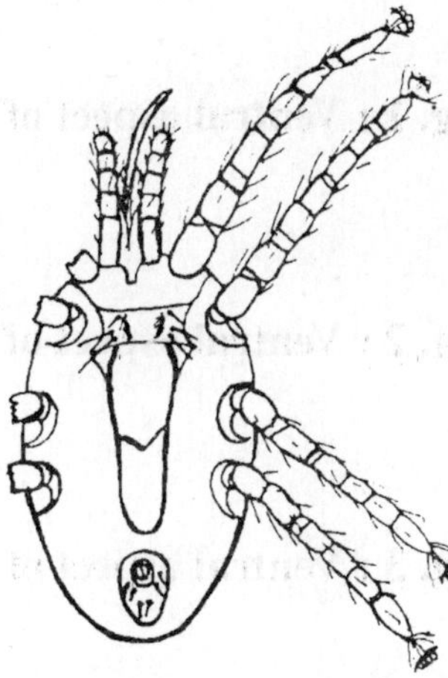

Fig. 2

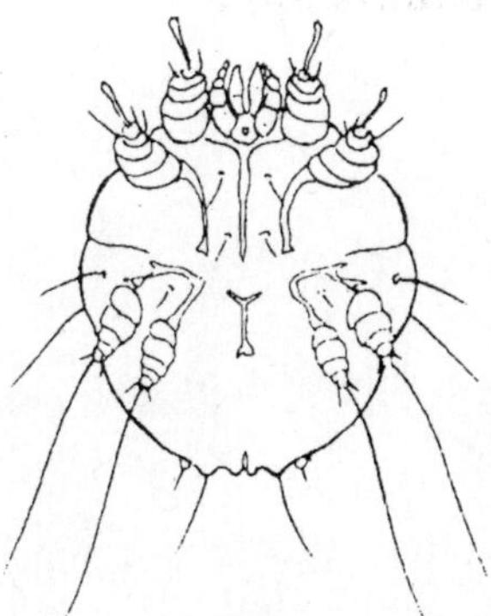

Fig. 3

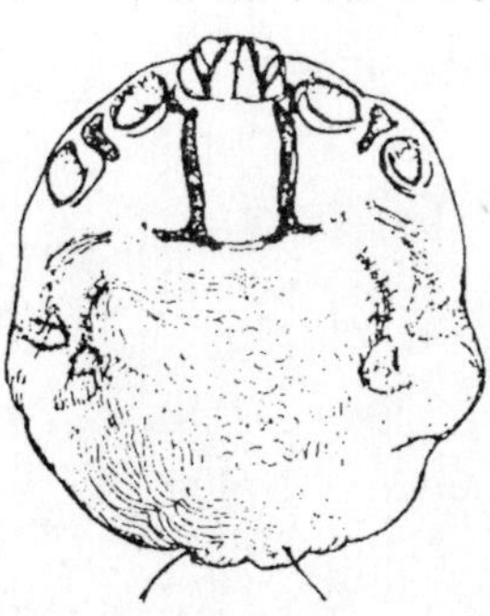

Fig. 4

PLATE XXIX

Fig. 1 : Ventral aspect of a male *Psoroptes ovis*

Fig. 2 : Ventral aspect of a male *Chorioptes bovis*

Fig. 3 : Ventral aspect of a female *Otodectes cynotis*

Fig. 4 : Ventral aspect of a male *Demodex folliculorum*

Fig. 5 : Dorsal aspect of *Leptotrombidium* spp.

PLATE XXIX

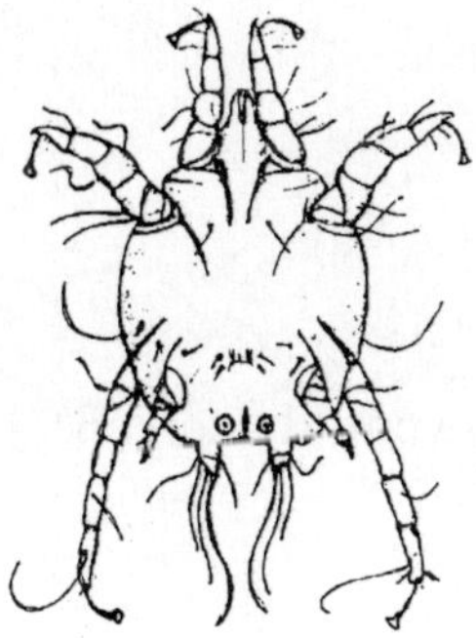

Fig. 1

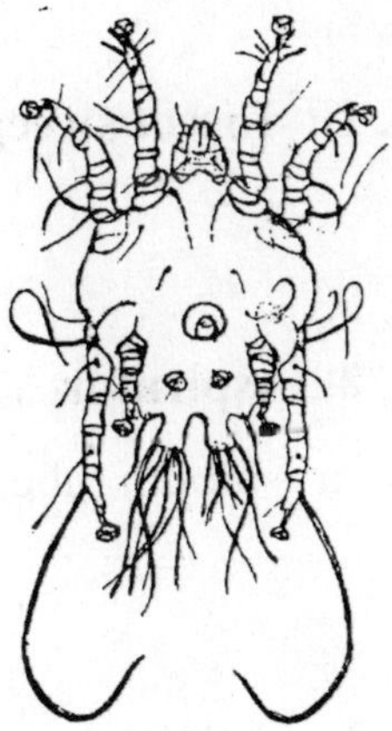

Fig. 2

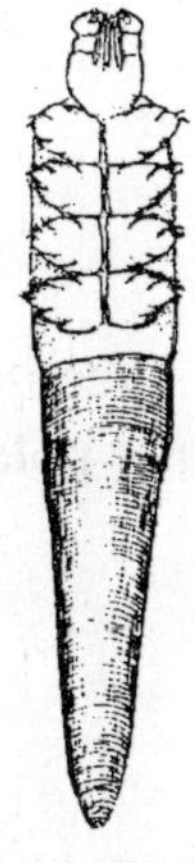

Fig. 4

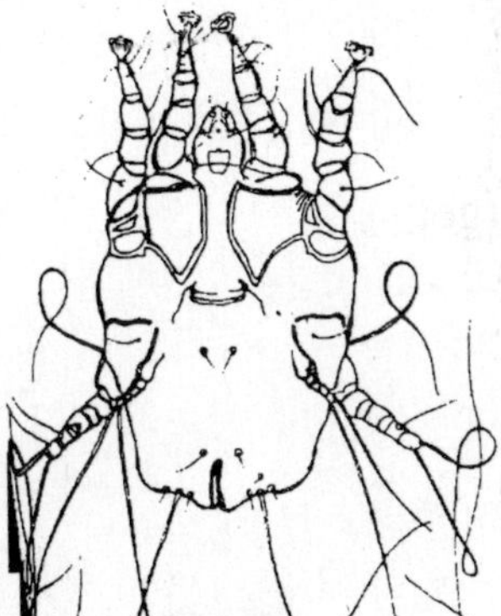

Fig. 3

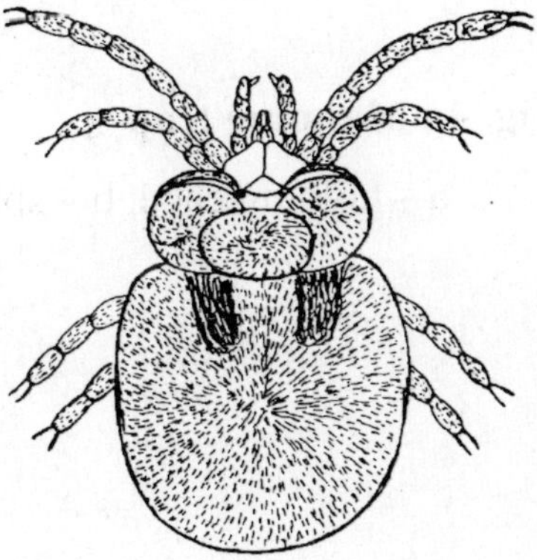

Fig. 5

PLATE XXX

Fig. 1 : Insect/sweeping net

Fig. 2 : Aspirator

a – mouth tube, b – entry tube, c – vent, d - screen

Fig. 3 : Malaise trap

a – holding cage, b – screen fabric, c – center pole, d – corner skirt, e – corner pole

Fig. 4 : Manning trap

a – holding cage, b – sphere target

PLATE XXX

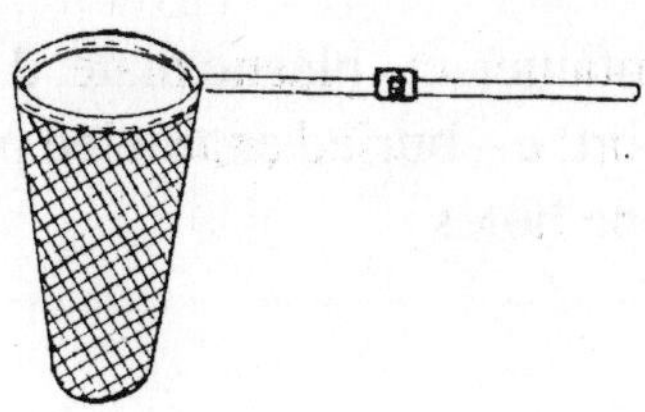

Fig. 1

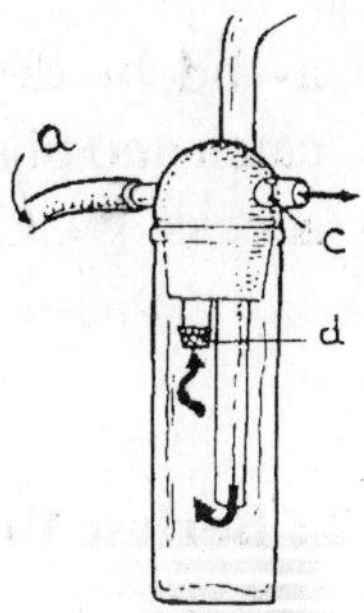

Fig. 2

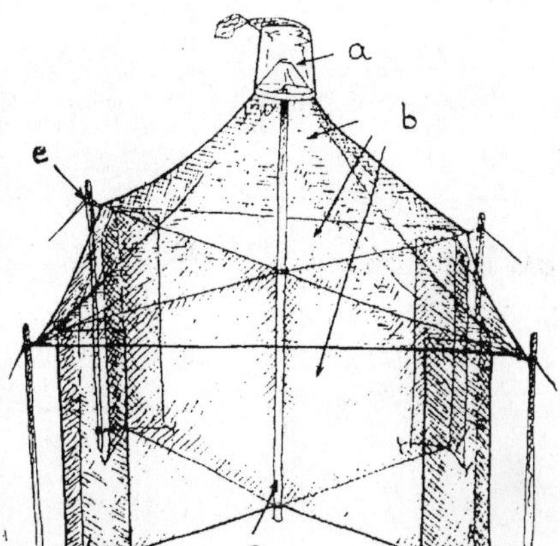

Fig. 3

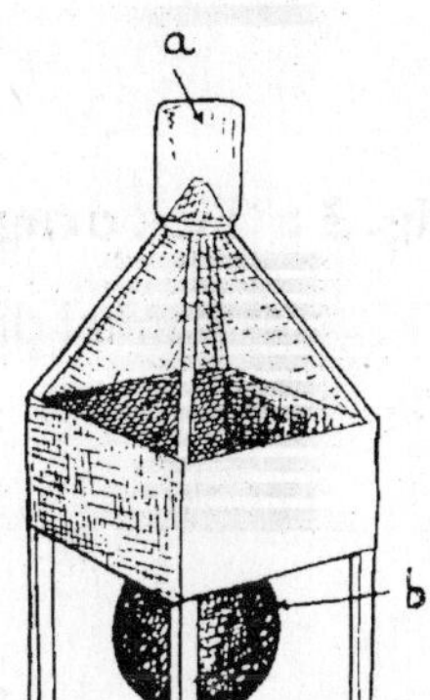

Fig. 4

PLATE XXXI

Fig. 1 : Dry ice/ Co_2 burrow trap

a – lid, b – dry ice container, c – plastic plate, d – moisture catch and plate support, e – buried enameled pan, f – tick access, g – Co_2 escape holes

Fig. 2 : Berlese funnel

a – lid, b – collecting jar, c – wire rack, d – sample, e – repellent or heat source

Fig. 3 : Tick drag

a – flannel drag, b – draw bar

PLATE XXXI

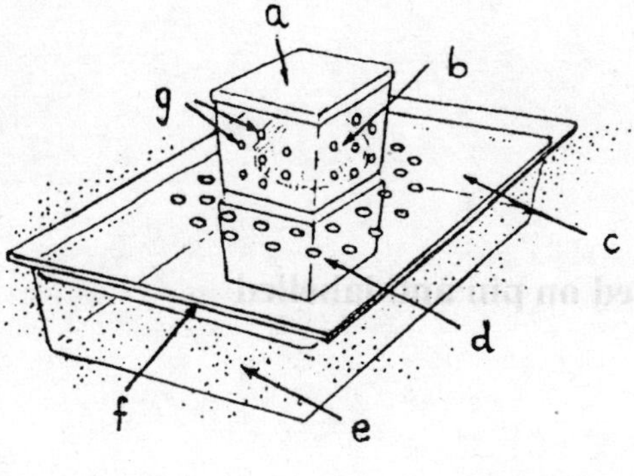

Fig. 1

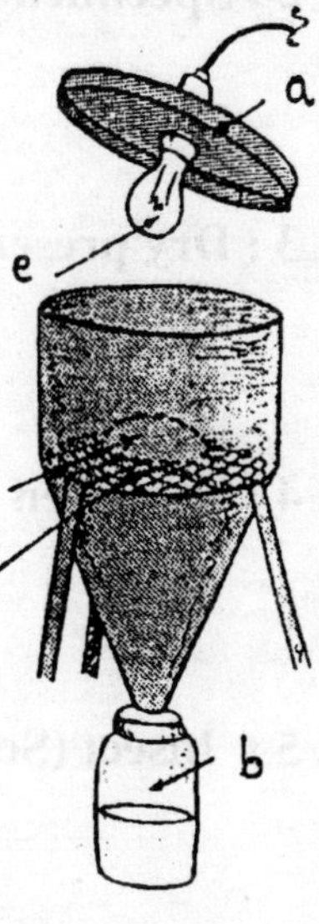

Fig. 2

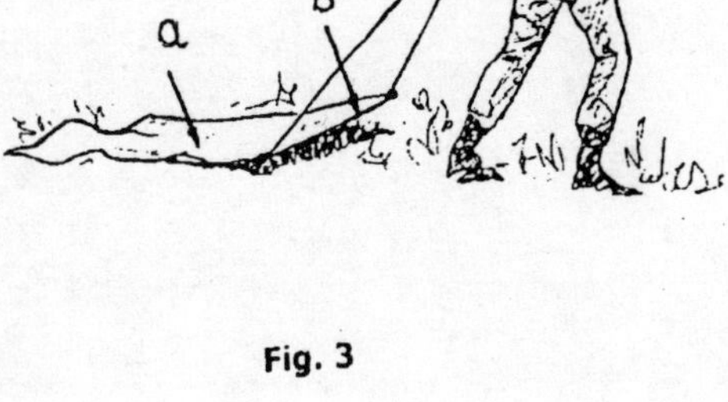

Fig. 3

PLATE XXXII

Fig. 1 : Insect killing jar

Fig. 2 : Specimen impaled on pin and labelled

Fig. 3 : Dry preservation of insects

Fig. 4 : Specimen on a small needle and cork block

Fig. 5 : Insect (Schmitt) box

PLATE XXXII

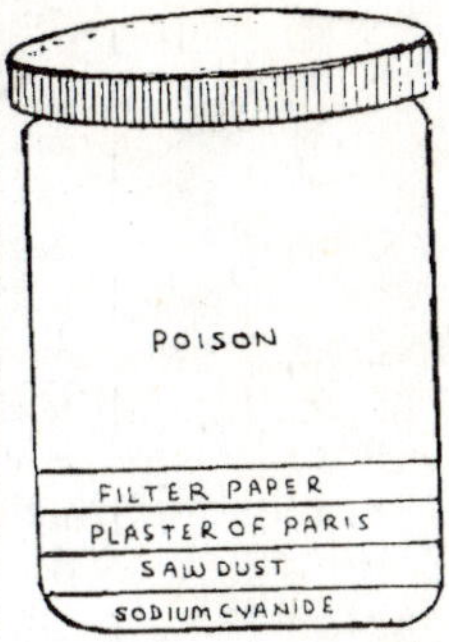

Fig. 1

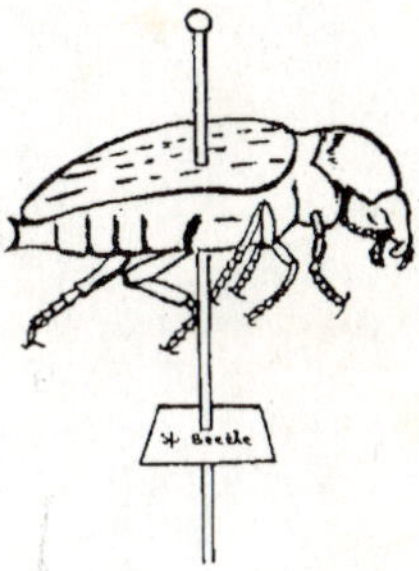

Fig. 2

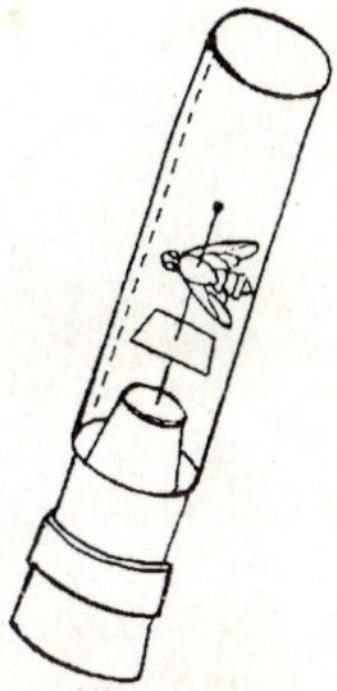

Fig. 3

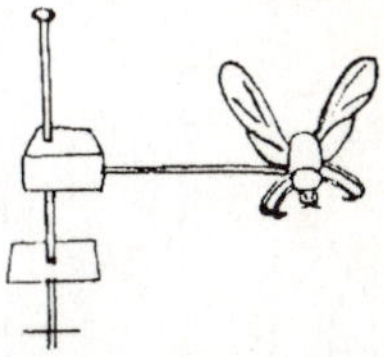

Fig. 4

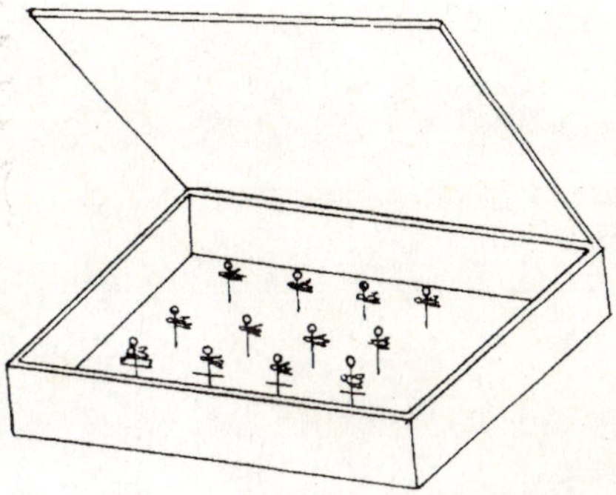

Fig. 5